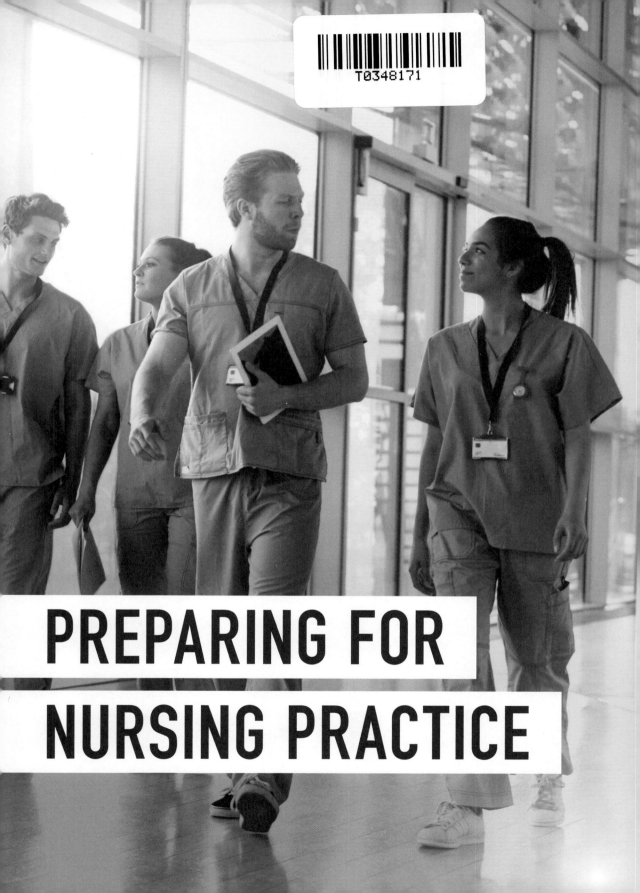

PREPARING FOR
NURSING PRACTICE

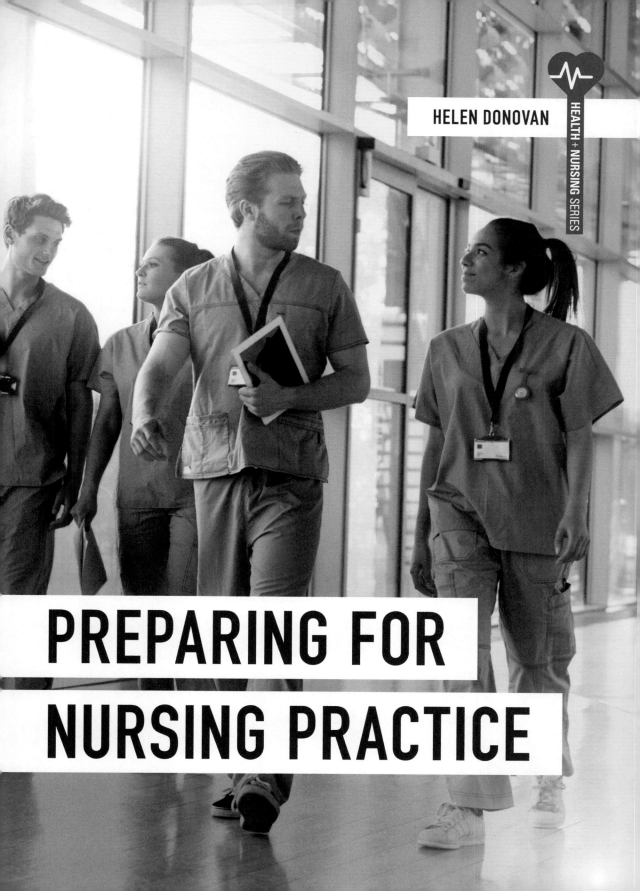

HELEN DONOVAN

HEALTH + NURSING SERIES

PREPARING FOR
NURSING PRACTICE

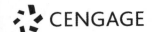
CENGAGE

Preparing for nursing practice
1st Edition
Helen Donovan

Product manager: Michelle Aarons
Content developer: Lynley Bidlake
Project editor: Alex Chambers
Project and cover designer: Mariana Maccarini
Text designer: Rina Gargano (Alba Design)
Editor: Sylvia Marson
Proofreader: Jade Jakovcic
Permissions/Photo researcher: Catherine Kerstjens
Indexer: Julie King
Cover: Shutterstock.com/Monkey Business Images
Typeset by KnowledgeWorks Global Ltd.

Any URLs contained in this publication were checked for
currency during the production process. Note, however, that
the publisher cannot vouch for the ongoing currency of URLs.

For product information and technology assistance,
in Australia call **1300 790 853**;
in New Zealand call **0800 449 725**

For permission to use material from this text or product, please email
aust.permissions@cengage.com

National Library of Australia Cataloguing-in-Publication Data
ISBN: 9780170460453
A catalogue record for this book is available from the National Library of
Australia.

Cengage Learning Australia
Level 5, 80 Dorcas Street
Southbank VIC 3006 Australia

Cengage Learning New Zealand
Unit 4B Rosedale Office Park
331 Rosedale Road, Albany, North Shore 0632, NZ

For learning solutions, visit **cengage.com.au**

Printed in China by 1010 Printing International Limited.
1 2 3 4 5 6 7 27 26 25 24 23

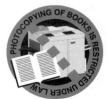

BRIEF CONTENTS

CONTENTS

PART 1   BEING PRACTICE READY   1

Guide to the text

As you read this text you will find a number of features in every chapter to enhance your study of nursing and help you understand how the theory is applied in the real world.

PART OPENING FEATURES

Part openers introduce each of the chapters within the part and give an overview of how they relate to each other.

CHAPTER OPENING FEATURES

Refer to the **Introduction** for an overview of the chapter.

Introduction

The mantra 'wherever there are people, there are nurses' provides you with a sense of the breadth of nursing-related positions available and offers you a starting point for where you may look for employment as a graduate registered nurse (GRN). Nursing has always provided a diversity of practice opportunities that also allow travel and flexibility around family commitments and postgraduate studies. You may think that planning your nursing career while a GRN is too early, but your career goals will take you to a place where you will celebrate your achievements, and it is your professional vision that guides your career journey. It is never too early to start thinking about your career and the environment in which you would like to live and work. Websites

Identify the key concepts you will engage with through the **Learning objectives** at the start of each chapter.

CHAPTER
4
PREPARING FOR A NEW HEALTH CARE ENVIRONMENT AS A GRN

Learning objectives

Working through this chapter will enable you to:

1. value the population trends that influence nursing employment opportunities in Australia
2. compare opportunities in different health care environments
3. incorporate health promotion and disease prevention into professional practice
4. visualise nursing opportunities within different contexts of care
5. understand how the National Health Priority Areas will be fundamental in your preparation for practice.

FEATURES WITHIN CHAPTERS

Examine how theoretical concepts can been used in practice through the **Reflection** boxes.

REFLECTION: THE CHANGING IMAGE OF THE NURSE

The global COVID-19 pandemic has demonstrated how a single virus can bring catastrophic changes on an international scale. The need for nursing care has never been greater and the thousands of images of nurses from every country in the world in full personal protective equipment (PPE) highlights the importance of this large workforce of health care professionals.

a   In your groups, discuss how the public image of nurses has changed globally.

b   Describe how nurses' public health roles expanded during the COVID-19 pandemic and how nurses

Engage actively and personally with the material by completing the practical activities in the **Practical application** boxes. These help you to assess your own knowledge, goals, traits and attitudes.

PRACTICAL APPLICATION: ADVOCACY

You are working in a busy surgical ward. It is your first night shift and your allocated preceptor has called in sick. When you observe the nursing team on the night shift, there are only two RNs, one is team leader and the other is a graduate with only three months more experience than yourself. The remainder of the staff are enrolled nurses. Your patient allocation has responsibilities that are outside of your scope of practice. You are aware that you are going to need to speak up so that you can have the workforce support you will need for the shift.

Discuss in small groups how you will:
•   advocate for yourself so that you have the adequate support to care for the patients you have

Analyse **Case studies** that present issues in context, encouraging you to integrate the concepts discussed in the chapter and apply them to the workplace.

CASE **STUDY**

HEALTH PROMOTION – EXAMPLE

An obese man, Jason, who is a long-term tobacco smoker with chronic asthma is admitted to the medical ward as he has a chest infection and is ordered intravenous antibiotic treatment. During the admission, Jason tells you that he does not wear his seatbelt when driving his car as he finds it too uncomfortable due to his current size. Thinking about this case study scenario, it is clear that Jason needs primary prevention support to wear his seat belt when driving in the car, secondary prevention support to address his obesity and tobacco use and tertiary prevention support to address his chronic asthma.

How did you go? boxes contain responses, prompts and tips for other activities.

HOW DID YOU GO?

If you said that you would prefer to work with RNs who demonstrate professional attitudes and behaviours, that is very common. People who work and act professionally are typically reliable, trustworthy and honest. Working with someone who displays a 'no care' attitude to your learning, who arrives late and unprepared for the shift and does not communicate professionally with you, is

FEATURES WITHIN CHAPTERS

Identify client health and safety issues and responses to critical situations with **Safety in nursing** boxes.

SAFETY IN NURSING

WORKPLACE SAFETY ISSUES

Draw a floor plan of the layout of your last placement. Include all areas that you can recall. Identify where workplace safety issues were of concern/or had the potential for concern during your

END-OF-CHAPTER FEATURES

At the end of each chapter you will find several tools to help you to review, practise and extend your knowledge of the key learning objectives.

Review your understanding of the key chapter topics with the **Summary**.

FOCUS POINTS AND MOVING FORWARD

The rapid changes in health care and the global trends of disease processes provides a fundamental repositioning of the nurse's scope of practice, employment and practice options. The need for changes in practice are also influenced by digital health records in Australia, which provide a national image of health care needs and services. It is the understanding of the health care environment from a broader scope that enables you, as an RN, to understand the trends and changes that are occurring in your own health care environment. This will assist you to prepare for changing needs in the population as a whole, which will mean changes in treatment plans and new equipment developed to improve care options.

DISCUSSION POINTS

1. Consider health care equipment that you have used in the clinical environment. Discuss how you ensured that the patient, rather than the health care equipment, was central to the

Extend your understanding with the **References** relevant to each chapter.

REFERENCES

Australian Institute of Health and Welfare. (2018). *Culturally and linguistically diverse populations. Australia's health 2018.* Australia's health series no. 16. AUS 221. Canberra: AIHW. https://www.aihw.gov.au/getmedia/f3ba8e92-afb3-46d6-b64c-ebfc9c1f945d/aihw-aus-221-chapter-5-3.pdf
Australian Institute of Health and Welfare (2021). *Health system overview.* https://www.aihw.gov.au/reports/australias-health/health-system-overview

Discover high-quality online educational resources to support your nursing practice in the **Useful weblinks** lists.

USEFUL WEBSITES

Australian Safety and Quality Framework for Health Care, https://www.safetyandquality.gov.au/sites/default/files/migrated/ASQFHC-Guide-Healthcare-team.pdf
Australian Institute of Health and Welfare (AIHW), Health system overview (updated 2021), https://www.aihw.gov.au/reports/australias-health/health-system-overview

Guide to the online resources

Cengage is pleased to provide you with a selection of resources that will help you prepare your lectures and assessments. These teaching tools are accessible via cengage.com.au/instructors for Australia or cengage.co.nz/instructors for New Zealand.

INSTRUCTOR'S MANUAL

The Instructor's manual includes:
- Learning objectives
- Suggested class discussions and projects
- And more

POWERPOINT™ PRESENTATIONS

Use the chapter-by-chapter **PowerPoint slides** to enhance your lecture presentations and handouts by reinforcing the key principles of your subject.

ARTWORK FROM THE TEXT

Add the **digital files** of tables, pictures and flow charts into your learning management system, use them in student handouts, or copy them into your lecture presentations.

BEING PRACTICE READY

Learning outcomes

1. Describe and explain what professional practice readiness looks like.
2. Value the opportunities of being a graduate registered nurse for personal and professional development.
3. Understand that the roles and responsibilities of a beginner registered nurse are a key to expanding your scope of practice.

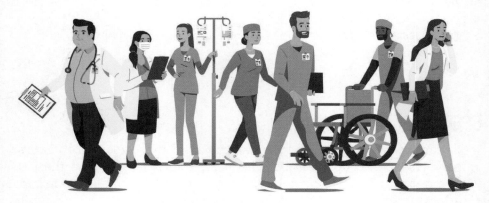

Source: Shutterstock.com/Iconic Bestiary

1 PROFESSIONAL PRACTICE READINESS

Learning objectives

Working through this chapter will enable you to:

1. validate the diversity of professional practice readiness for the beginning registered nurse
2. value the importance of working within professional boundaries to facilitate and demonstrate practice readiness
3. recognise and explore professional practice issues that may influence practice readiness for the graduate registered nurse
4. display confidence in your knowledge and abilities in professional settings.

Introduction

Being 'practice ready' is a phrase that was coined in the 1970s and can be seen in Kramer's (1974) text *Reality Shock. Why nurses leave nursing* where the phrase 'hitting the ground running' was noted to be an expectation of all RNs regardless of education background. At that stage, the meaning was intentionally focused on the graduate nurse being expected to have the practiced skills of an experienced registered nurse (RN). Outcries that the graduate registered nurse's (GRN's) clinical skills were not adequate for practice were countered by others advocating for a reasoned approach, arguing that expecting the university educated RNs to have the same clinical exposure as the hospital trained RNs of the time was not reasonable and not workable (Greenwood, 2000).

Contemporary professional practice readiness for GRNs has been repositioned, with industry partners looking for graduates who bring professional behaviours and attitudes (soft science skills) to their GRN roles and responsibilities. These include those of effective communication, critical thinking and problem solving skills. This chapter explores how you, as a GRN, can work safely and confidently within your scope of practice, where you not only provide safe person-centered care, but also feel safe and confident in your practice role.

1.1 What does professional practice look like for the GRN?

Professional nursing practice is a highly regulated profession, that is guided by a discipline specific knowledge base and a unique Code of Ethics (2021) (see Figure 1.1). Behaviours, attitudes and expectations are described and regulated by the Nursing and Midwifery Board of Australia's (NMBA) Codes of conduct and Standards for practice. These standards are predominantly in place to protect the public; however, they are also used to assess students of nursing and to determine if care provided is within legal and ethical expectations of practice and that the student is ready to practice as an RN. As a GRN, your beginner status does not exempt you from working as a professional RN, but it does afford you the considerations that you are a beginner who will need guidance and **support**.

professional nursing practice
Nursing practice that is within the regulatory body's expectations of practice.

support
Assistance that is provided to ensure that nurses can meet their responsibilities.

While you may enter your first position as an RN with concerns that you are not prepared to care for patients independently, you should be reassured that you were assessed against the NMBA's professional standards for practice via the Australian Nursing Standards Assessment Tool (ANSAT). To have been assessed as satisfactory in all zones of the tool demonstrates that you have been working at a professional level, and it was determined that you have the capability to do so as a beginning RN.

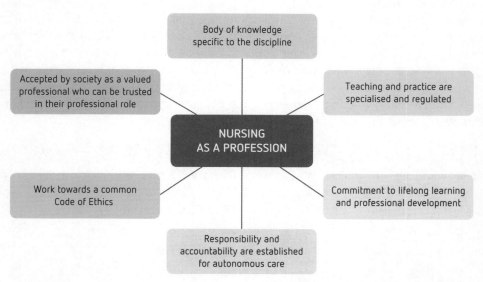

Adapted from Black, 2019; Kearney-Nunnery, 2020.

▶ Figure 1.1   Fundamental concepts of nursing as a profession

Working within your scope of practice to be professional practice ready

One of the more significant changes for you when first working as a GRN is that you must be able to independently determine and confidently state and work within your **scope of practice**. This provision ensures that all patients receive care that is based in nursing knowledge and clinical skills that are commensurate with safe practice (see also Figure 1.2).

As a student, your scope of practice was predetermined by your course progression. As a GRN you need to have the **confidence** to not only know the limits of your scope of practice but to seek assistance and direction when care needs fall outside of your **competencies**. You must then effectively utilise these experiences to develop and grow your expertise and expand your scope of practice towards that of an expert nurse. For some GRNs, identifying their scope of practice is seen as a daunting task, with graduates known to seek help from other RNs in their decision making. It is, however, only you who can make the decision as to the breadth of your scope of practice. It is only you who knows the level of your knowledge and clinical skills as well as your level of competence and confidence when implementing those skills or making clinical decisions that ensure safe practice.

From a professional practice position, attempting to provide care that is outside of your scope of practice is regarded as unprofessional behaviour, and as the RN you would be accountable for the outcome of the care provided. If you sought suitable assistance or guidance to safely implement the task, you would then be working within professional guidelines. Therefore, there is no expectation for you to know everything. The expectation is that you will provide person-centered care that sits within the NMBA's standards and policies of practice and within your capabilities. If you would like to read more about practice decisions in relation to scope of practice, review the Decision-making framework for nursing and midwifery (see the list of useful websites at the end of the chapter).

scope of practice
The extent of a nurse's ability to provide care based on their level of education and experience.

confidence
A sense of knowing that your judgement is correct and accurate.

competency
Meeting expected benchmarks.

Scope of practice	
Nursing knowledge and confidence in practice	**Clinical experience and ability to apply theory to practice**
Educational preparation	Clinical decision making
Legal position to practice	Holistic person-centered care
Knowledge to make clinical decisions	Context of care
Clinical experience and skills level	Support structures and personnel
Ability to apply theoretical knowledge to practice	Pre-determined goals

▶ Figure 1.2 Determining your scope of practice

Professional behaviours and attitudes

Industry partners are expressing a preference for GRNs who enter the profession displaying high levels of professionalism in the form of **professional attitudes** and behaviours towards nursing practice. Points of contention, such as graduates not presenting on time for their shift, not wearing the correct uniform and being indifferent to patient needs, have been identified as concerns from industry partners. These behaviours depict attitudes that do not value or embrace professional expectations. In essence, your attitudes are the cognitive processes behind your behaviours, and are showcased by your efforts to work to the professional standards of nursing practice, your response to feedback, and how you communicate and collaborate with the **health care team** (Masters, 2018; Masters & Gilmore, 2018). All aspects of your **professional behaviours** and attitudes are reflective of your professional **practice readiness**.

professional attitude
An attitude that exhibits the regulatory body's expectations when working as a professional registered nurse.

health care team
All members of a team of health care professionals.

professional behaviour
Behaviours that exhibit the regulatory body's expectations when working as a professional registered nurse.

practice readiness
Having the knowledge and skills to practice as a registered nurse.

REFLECTION: EMBRACING PROFESSIONAL PRACTICE ATTITUDES AND BEHAVIOURS IN NURSING

In a small group:
a   Describe and list the characteristics of RNs who you felt demonstrated professional attitudes and behaviours during your clinical placement.
b   List the characteristics of those RNs who you felt demonstrated unprofessional attitudes and behaviours during your clinical placement.
c   Discuss how the differences in professional attitudes and behaviours of RNs impacted your ability, and the opportunity, to learn in the clinical environment as a student of nursing.
d   Discuss how you anticipate working with RNs who demonstrate professional behaviour will support you as a GRN in your professional development and the expansion of your scope of practice.
     After your discussions, create and complete a table like the example below.

Professional attitudes and enabling behaviours	Unprofessional attitudes and limiting behaviours

HOW DID YOU GO?

If you said that you would prefer to work with RNs who demonstrate professional attitudes and behaviours, that is very common. People who work and act professionally are typically reliable, trustworthy and honest. Working with someone who displays a 'no care' attitude to your learning, who arrives late and unprepared for the shift and does not communicate professionally with you, is not only a barrier to your learning but to the team as a whole. Keep this in mind when you are working as an RN in the health care sector.

Using your clinical placement experiences to develop professional practice readiness

Your clinical placement experiences are integral for you to learn and develop professional behaviours and attitudes. Approaching clinical placement from a position of strength, where you have the knowledge and understanding of the profession of nursing and the legal, moral and ethical expectations behind the profession, places you in a strong position where you are able work within those standards, guidelines and policies of practice under the guidance of other RNs. If you enter clinical placement having limited understanding of these expectations, it will place you in a position of vulnerability.

As a student, you may have found that some people in your care are very supportive of your learning and are understanding and tolerant of time delays due to you needing to obtain support and supervision. Others may have been less positive to the point where they voice their frustration. Your response to any situation must be measured, empathic and culturally safe with an overarching aim to enable the therapeutic relationship to be maintained at all times (O'Toole, 2020). With the support from your buddy nurse and facilitators, you will be able to seek advice and observe how others work through difficult or complex situations. In essence, you are developing your own ability to work professionally in uncertain circumstances when immersed in these experiences. Work through the following case study to reinforce how you should respond to a challenging situation.

CASE **STUDY**

RESPONDING IN A CHALLENGING SITUATION

You are working as a student of nursing in a busy general surgical unit in a regional hospital. A 24-year-old male patient, Josh, has returned from the operating theatre two hours previously after an elective tonsillectomy. You notice fresh blood in his nasal cavity, and he appears to be swallowing regularly and complaining of pain. Josh's vital signs are all within normal range; however, you feel that he is quieter than he was earlier and is refusing to suck the ice you provided for him, saying that 'it doesn't help'. Josh's mother is present and wants to know if the pain Josh is experiencing is normal and she is worried that he appears to be agitated and doesn't seem to be responding to her when she speaks to him. She asks if you should get the RN to help you.

a   In pairs, discuss what may be the cause of Josh's mother's distress. Also discuss why you should take all concerns raised by family members seriously.

b   Under the headings of 'Open communication', 'Therapeutic relationship' and 'Scope of practice', describe how you would respond to Josh's mother's concerns.

Open communication	Therapeutic relationship	Scope of practice

HOW DID YOU GO?

Did you understand how open communication, honesty and active listening enhances the therapeutic relationship? Did you see how working within your scope of practice to confidently provide safe care, but then seeking assistance when the clinical situation was outside of your scope of practice, ensured that both the patient and you were safe, and you could reassure Josh's mother?

1.2 Practice readiness and professional boundaries

In situations such as the example scenario in the case study, it can be a challenge for both the student nurse and the GRN to stay within their boundaries of professional practice (Black, 2019). **Professional boundaries** are invisible borders of practice aimed to protect both you and the person in your care. The main goal is to provide care that is central to the person's needs – this is a therapeutic relationship; that is, a helpful relationship. If the relationship is no longer person-centred and becomes about the nurse and their needs, then the professional boundary has been crossed (NMBA, 2020). For example, an overly attentive (or involved) nurse may be working outside of professional boundaries, by seeking a personal rather than a professional connection with a patient. Whereas an under-attentive nurse who ignores or dismisses a patient's

professional boundaries
Invisible borders of practice aimed to protect both you and the person in your care.

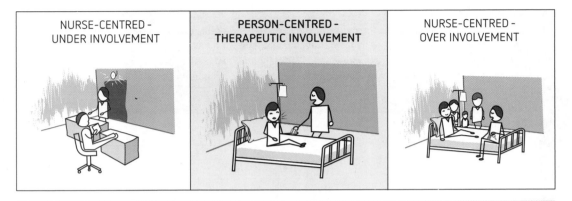

| NURSE-CENTRED –
UNDER INVOLVEMENT | PERSON-CENTRED –
THERAPEUTIC INVOLVEMENT | NURSE-CENTRED –
OVER INVOLVEMENT |

▶ **Figure 1.3** Working within professional boundaries ensures that the nurse provides care that is person-centred and therapeutic

needs in preference to their own, while also regarded to be working outside of professional boundaries, is said to be working from a position of under-involvement of the person's care (see Figure 1.3). Difficulties in professional boundaries can also arise when a patient seeks out a personal relationship, such as asking to join a nurse's Facebook page, or asking for their personal phone number. The nurse must draw the relationship back into the therapeutic zone without offending or embarrassing the patient. Being aware of what person-centred care and a therapeutic relationship looks like is essential for the GRN to know when professional boundaries are crossed and also how the boundary can be reinstated back to the therapeutic zone of helpfulness. Working with the NMBA's Code of conduct and social media guidelines will provide you with the reassurance you may need to work in these challenging situations (see the list of useful websites at the end of the chapter).

Using humour to maintain professional boundaries

Many nurses find that humour is a valuable tool to use; for example, to deflect an inappropriate suggestion as a joke or as a cryptic comment that can't be taken seriously. It is difficult though, and it takes experience to confidently respond with empathy, professionalism and lighthearted humour so that the therapeutic relationship can be maintained and the professional boundary kept intact. Along with Section 4.1 Professional boundaries of the NMBA's Code of conduct and the Australian College of Nursing's publication *Maintaining professional boundaries* (ACN, 2020), there are many valuable resources with examples and case studies that highlight and clarify situations where professional boundaries may have the potential to be crossed. These resources will provide you with examples on how to respond in these difficult circumstances and how you can retain your professionalism.

1.3. Practice readiness and professional practice issues

Issues with professional practice can lead to significant concerns and distress for all involved. Issues that are commonly shared are those that relate to the workforce and to the workplace and these ultimately impact on the provision of safe patient care.

Workforce issues

Workforce issues are those that occur from a workforce position. They may include issues of communication breakdowns, or where the skill mix between staff does not enable safe or effective patient care, or it may relate to staff shortages where the workload cannot be met due to a limited number of staff. All nurses have a responsibility to identify workforce issues, so that patient care is not hindered or lacking. For the GRN, a lack of support due to workforce issues has the potential for them to work outside of their scope of practice, and if care is impacted as a result, can lead to a **conflict** situation.

workforce issues
Situations that occur within the workforce; for example, communication breakdowns or staff shortages.

conflict
A situation where there is a misunderstanding or misinterpretation of a message.

Conflict and bullying behaviours in the workforce

Conflict and **bullying** are noted to often be the result of workforce issues, when communication breakdowns or unreasonable expectations are made of the GRN. While the terms are often used interchangeably, their meaning and intention in the clinical area and impact on the graduate can be quite different. It is important to clarify this as responses to each situation are quite different (see Figure 1.4).

bullying
A situation where a person or group of people cause repeated and intentional harm to another.

Conflict can be the result of a difference of opinion or a different perspective to a situation (Henderson, 2019). It is primarily seen as a misunderstanding or misinterpretation of a situation, and with reasoned discussion can easily be overcome. It is understood to be unintentional, and all people involved will work collaboratively to resolve the confusion.

Bullying behaviours, however, are those that are intentional and repeated, with a purpose to injure, undermine or intimidate a person, and to generally cause harm and destabilise the person (O'Toole, 2020).

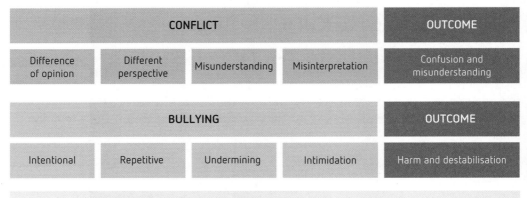

▶ Figure 1.4   Behaviours seen in conflict and bullying situations

Both conflict and bullying situations can delay practice readiness by limiting professional practice opportunities and causing undue confusion and an overall lack of confidence. The experience of conflict, however, can also enhance the GRN's preparation for practice, as they learn to navigate and work with situations where behaviours of the health care team (and people in their care) may be challenging or combative.

It is essential that GRNs can confidently clarify language and behaviours to ensure that messages are not misconstrued and to limit the escalation to a damaging experience. Sometimes the GRN who has worked to clarify a situation and to understand the person's behaviours, may find that support from their supervisor, **educator** or preceptor may be needed. Refer to the 'Bullying and harassment' section of the NMBA's Code of conduct for nurses (p. 10) to assist in clarifying and understanding expectations in relation to safe professional behaviours, and in recognising and responding to experiences of conflict, bullying and harassment.

educator
A person who provides information and learning.

Workplace issues

workplace issues
Situations in the work environment that impact on the ability of a nurse to practice professionally.

Workplace issues are those that relate to the environment in which you work. The workplace does include the workforce, but ultimately it is about how you perceive or interpret the environment around you and whether it impacts on your ability to practice professionally (Assi et al., 2019). Workplace issues can be as obvious as water on the ground that constitutes a slip hazard, a lack of equipment in which to provide adequate care, or a lack of support in the form of policies and procedures. As a GRN, you have a responsibility to identify any workplace issues and report those to your immediate supervisor. It is important to understand what your roles and responsibilities are when addressing workplace issues. For example, you would be expected to independently remove the spilled water from the ground, but a lack of equipment or broken equipment would need to be reported to your team leader who will escalate the issue. Policy and procedure issues also need to be escalated through the correct channels, so you will to need understand what these are before moving forward.

1.4. Confidence and practice readiness

Confidence is an expected characteristic of all GRNs. It is important to understand that being confident does not mean that you know everything. Being confident is being positive about what you do know and what you don't know. For example, it is essential that you are aware of your scope of practice and are confident in what clinical skills you can undertake independently and what skills you need assistance with. It is also essential that you are able to confidently identify when you do not have the knowledge and clinical decision-making experience to make a safe clinical decision. Confidence also extends to your interactions with other health care professionals, where you have the confidence to share your knowledge and understanding of a patient's health care needs in the collaborative setting (Caballero & Walker, 2021). This collaboration needs to be from a position of working within your scope of practice and always using professional language and collaborative processes.

Reflecting to develop confidence and competence

A reflective approach to practice provides you with the opportunity to draw from an experience and learn from those events and interactions. Reflection is a professional expectation of all RNs and is an essential approach to practice that allows you to grow and develop your expertise as a nurse. The greater the depth of your exploration and reasoning about a situation, the more understanding and insight you will gain. To guide your reflective practices, there are many different frameworks, but ultimately you should work with the one that makes the most sense to you. Complete the following reflection activity to see how much depth of understanding and reasoning you gained from a previous experience.

REFLECTION: USING REFLECTION TO DEVELOP YOUR PROFESSIONALISM

Write reflective paragraphs based on the following scenario.

a   Describe a situation when you were very disappointed in someone or something during your clinical placement.

b   Describe exactly what made you feel disappointed and if your reaction was a surprise to you. Why wasn't your response one of anger or frustration?

c   Describe if your reaction impacted on your ability to respond professionally.

d   Describe how you would respond if this situation were to happen again.
    Discuss your response with your classmates to gauge their perception of your response.

HOW DID YOU GO?

Reflection is not always easy and it can take some time to delve deeply into an experience. For example, you may have felt that the other person didn't behave as expected, that your position was not considered, or that what happened didn't fit with your plan. Now think about why you weren't angry or sad or happy with the outcomes, but disappointed instead. It is asking these types of questions that will help you to unearth what was behind your response so that you can move forward with a greater understanding of how you see the world and how you react in certain circumstances. This level of exploration will often lead you to initiate change in your professional attitude or behaviours, so that you can confidently move forward in your practice.

FOCUS POINTS AND MOVING FORWARD

Professional practice in nursing is a fundamental expectation that enables effective and safe patient care. As a graduate, your professionalism has been influenced by the knowledge and experiences that you have gained and is guided by the codes and frameworks of the regulatory bodies of practice. Ultimately, your professional practice readiness will be guided by your intrinsic desire to work as a safe and motivated RN who strives for best practice. Seeing yourself in this 'light' is central to not only your professional development but to your identity as an effective and efficient RN.

DISCUSSION POINTS

1. Discuss how clearly stating that you are working within your scope of practice demonstrates professionalism to your colleagues.

    _____

    _____

    _____

    _____

2. Reflect on a challenging situation with a patient or their family that you experienced during your clinical placement. Discuss how you maintained professionalism and ensured that the therapeutic relationship was maintained.

    _____

    _____

    _____

    _____

3. Think about a time when you misunderstood an RN's instructions when you were a student of nursing. How did you ensure that you clarified the instruction so that the patient received safe care?

    _____

    _____

    _____

    _____

REFERENCES

Assi, M., Peterson, C., & Hatmaker, D. (2019). Workforce advocacy for professional nursing practice environment. In B. Cherry & S. Jacob (Eds.), *Contemporary nursing. Issues, trends and management* (8th ed., pp. 232–250). Elsevier.

Australian College of Nursing. (2020). *Maintaining professional boundaries.* https://www.acn.edu.au/wp-content/uploads/career-hub-resources-maintaining-professional-boundaries.pdf

Black, B. (2019). *Professional nursing: concepts and challenges* (9th ed.) Elsevier.

Caballero, C., & Walker, A. (2021). Industry readiness. In H. Harrison, M. Birks, and J. Mills (Eds.), *Transition to nursing practice. From student to professional* (pp. 200–216). Oxford University Press.

Greenwood, J. (2000). Critique of the graduate nurse: an international perspective. *Nurse Education Today, 20*(1), 17–23.

Henderson, A. (2019). *Communication for health care practice.* Oxford University Press.

Kearney-Nunnery, R. (2020). *Advancing your career – concepts of professional nursing.* FA Davis Company.

Kramer, M. (1974). *Reality Shock. Why nurses leave nursing.* C.V. Mosby Co.

Masters, K. (2018). Teamwork, collaboration and communication in professional nursing practice. In K. Masters (Ed.), *Role development in professional nursing practice* (5th ed., pp. 535–562). Jones & Bartlett Learning, LLC.

Masters, K., & Gilmore, M. (2018). Education and socialization to the professional nursing role. In K. Masters (Ed.), *Role development in professional nursing practice* (5th ed., pp. 219–241). Jones & Bartlett Learning, LLC.

Nursing and Midwifery Board of Australia. (2020). *Decision-making framework – nursing.* https://www.nursingmidwiferyboard.gov.au/codes-guidelines-statements/frameworks.aspx

O'Toole, G. (2020). *Communication. Core Interpersonal skills for healthcare professionals.* Elsevier.

USEFUL WEBSITES

Nursing and Midwifery Board of Australia, Code of conduct for nurses, https://www.nursingmidwiferyboard.gov.au/codes-guidelines-statements/professional-standards.aspx

Nursing and Midwifery Board of Australia, Decision-making framework – nursing and midwifery, https://www.nursingmidwiferyboard.gov.au/codes-guidelines-statements/frameworks.aspx

Nursing and Midwifery Board of Australia, Code of ethics, https://www.nursingmidwiferyboard.gov.au/codes-guidelines-statements/professional-standards.aspx

Nursing and Midwifery Board of Australia, Registered nurse standards for practice, https://www.nursingmidwiferyboard.gov.au/Codes-Guidelines-Statements/Professional-standards/registered-nurse-standards-for-practice.aspx

Nursing and Midwifery Board of Australia – Social media: How to meet your obligations under the National Law, https://www.ahpra.gov.au/Resources/Social-media-guidance.aspx

Australian College of Nursing, Career Hub, Maintaining Professional Boundaries, https://www.acn.edu.au/wp-content/uploads/career-hub-resources-maintaining-professional-boundaries.pdf

2 IDENTITY CHANGE AND ITS IMPLICATIONS FOR PERSONAL AND PROFESSIONAL DEVELOPMENT

Learning objectives

Working through this chapter will enable you to:

1. recognise internal and external influences on personal identity
2. recognise imposter syndrome and its potential to have a negative impact on your professional identity
3. understand how role change and role stress influences your perception of self
4. demonstrate how working with a collaborative team assists to manage role stress
5. recognise how lifelong learning can facilitate a resilient and confident approach to practice
6. understand how emotional literacy assists a resilient approach to practice.

Introduction

Even though you may have envisaged yourself as a registered nurse (RN) many times, it is not until you are working in an RN role that changes in professional expectations become a reality. Learning to present your new RN self to others as someone who is able to make clinical decisions and provide safe care is important for you to gain a sense of your changing identity. This chapter explores the role and professional identity change for the graduate RN (GRN) from the position of being a lifelong learner who draws from the collaborative team to ensure professional growth.

2.1. Personal identity: perceptions and expectations

Your personal **identity** offers you purpose and meaning in how you see yourself and the life you lead. This could be your physical, psychological or social self. How people identify themselves can be influenced by many factors. Physically, some people may see themselves as overweight, underweight or average weight, or tall or short. They may

identity
How a person sees themselves. A person's identify gives purpose and meaning in their life.

personal identity
How a person sees themselves in their everyday non-professional role.

also see their cognitive abilities as smart or average, and their social position as being employed or employable. Others may see themselves in a more negative light, as moody or hard to get along with. How others see you can influence how you see yourself as well. It is the balance of how you see yourself as a person and how others see you that will influence your perception of self and influence your **personal identity** (Gulliya, 2012). Frameworks such as the Johari Window are valuable when considering how your identity is perceived by not only yourself but by others (see Figure 2.1).

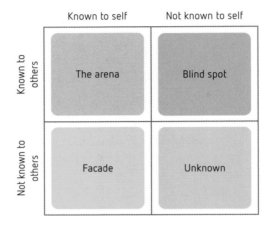

Source: Luft, J. & Ingham, H. (1955). 'The Johari window, a graphic model of interpersonal awareness'. Proceedings of the Western Training Laboratory in Group Development. Los Angeles: UCLA.

▶ **Figure 2.1** The Johari Window

Societal perceptions and identity change

change
A movement from one state to another. To transition into a different way of life.

Personal relationships can also **change** and shape a person's identity. Often there are societal expectations around how people will identify themselves; for example, as a single person or as someone in a relationship. Societal expectations and perceptions can be problematic, leading to some people being discriminated against or being seen as less valuable than other people. For example, one profession may be regarded as more important than another, or someone who drives a certain brand of car may be considered more affluent or important than a person who drives a less expensive car.

Societal expectations and perceptions can, however, be valuable for RNs. For example, nurses and the nursing profession are well-regarded and trusted by the general public in Australia. Therefore, when a person first seeks assistance from a nurse, they will enter the relationship with a sense of trust and acceptance of the nurse as a professional who can provide safe care. It would be much more difficult for a nurse to develop a therapeutic relationship with a patient, if the patient entered the relationship with a sense of doubt and scepticism.

2.2 Professional identity: perceptions and expectations

Your personal identity is the foundational layer of your perception of yourself as a professional. For example, you may identify as someone who is curious and outgoing. Your **professional identity** places another contextual layer of meaning over these identities. How you see yourself and how others see you in the professional world moves you towards your professional identity (Alexander & Stewart, 2020). For example, as a nursing student, you had the opportunity to receive constructive feedback in all stages of your bachelor program. This feedback would have reassured you of what you already knew about yourself, both personally and professionally, and would have provided information about things you didn't know about yourself that led you to further reflection.

professional identity
How a person sees themselves in their professional role.

Your professional identity is therefore multifaceted, and as a nurse it is the perceptions and assessment of yourself and that of others that will influence your sense of purpose, acceptance, belonging and control within the clinical environment (Black, 2019). Identity shifts are also influenced by the culture of the health care facility, the clinical expectations of the profession, and the acceptance by other health care professionals of you as a competent and trustworthy practitioner.

REFLECTION: REFLECTING ON YOUR IDENTITY

a   List the three top elements of how you identify yourself as a person (i.e. non-professional), a student of nursing and a GRN.
b   Look at the similarities and differences between each list and then create a flow chart that shows the strategies that you used to move between the 'person' identity to the 'student of nursing' when first entering nursing study, and then how you might move from the 'student of nursing' identity to the 'GRN' identity using similar strategies.

	Person	Strategies	Student	Strategies	GRN
ID elements					

Imposter syndrome

In the early stages of being a GRN, you may subconsciously still see yourself as a student, but consciously know that you are now an RN. So, one part of you knows that you are in the more autonomous role of being an RN, but the other is drawing you back to the more 'familiar' zone of being a student. You may find it all quite surreal, and struggle to believe that you are truly an RN. This uncertainty and disbelief in your position is often called **imposter syndrome**.

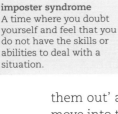

imposter syndrome
A time where you doubt yourself and feel that you do not have the skills or abilities to deal with a situation.

Impostor syndrome for GRNs is often reported in the early stages of the transition period (the first 1–3 months) and occurs when GRNs feel that they are working in a role they do not deserve or are unqualified to hold. Graduates have used the term 'pretending', saying they feel as though they are pretending to be an RN, and someone will 'catch them out' and expose them as a fraud. As a beginning RN, you may be struggling to move into the zone of being a GRN and working with the autonomy expected of you.

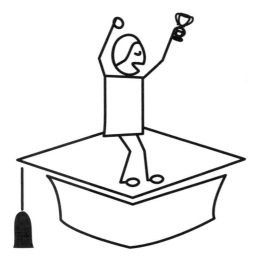

It is this instability of reasoning where you can sabotage your own effective transition to practice.

Be aware that impostor syndrome can be influenced by the expectations and support of those around you. If you are embraced as a graduate in your clinical area, with acknowledgement that your beginner foundational knowledge and skills are fertile grounds in which to grow into an expert nurse, then you will feel that you are legitimately working at the level of practice that aligns with your scope of practice. If your environment is one where you feel as though you are not meeting expectations, then that can undermine your confidence (Khan, 2021).

It is important as a GRN, therefore, to remember that you have studied and worked hard to gain your registration, and that you have been rigorously assessed against national standards of practice to achieve your registration. You were also appointed to the role after a thorough application and interview process. Holding the position is not one of chance. It is reflective of your knowledge and hard work to become the RN that you want to become.

2.3 Embracing change as a GRN

The ability to embrace change is central to the GRN's transition to practice journey. While some graduates may choose to accept positions in facilities where they had placement experiences, others will not. Either way there will be change. Some roles may be more complex and disruptive of previous routines and expectations, in other roles the change is not so obvious. Resisting or fighting against the change is not productive and will leave you feeling as though you have lost control of your professional and personal life.

Learning how to work with the new experiences you gain as a GRN will enable you to work towards your career goals and professional development aims. Emotionally healthy responses, such as being aware of how you respond to situations, manage stress and take care of your physical health and wellbeing are fundamental in finding purpose and meaning in your endeavours as a GRN (Purushothaman, 2021). This exploration provides a conduit in which to work towards accepting your identity change as a positive move forward to becoming the RN that you want to be.

Role change

The changing roles and responsibilities for GRNs are addressed more closely in Chapter 3 of this textbook; however, it is these changes that shape the beginning RN's perception of their professional identity. While many of the expectations remain the same as for a student of nursing, such as working within codes of conduct and ethics and within standards for practice, it is the lack of having a buddy nurse or a preceptor always supervising and overseeing them that graduates report to be the most concerning for them.

REFLECTION: PREPARING FOR PRACTICE

Create a concept map like the one shown below. In the top half of each cell list the knowledge and skills you gained as a student of nursing. Then, in the bottom half, write the knowledge and skills that you will need as a GRN working in the health care sector.

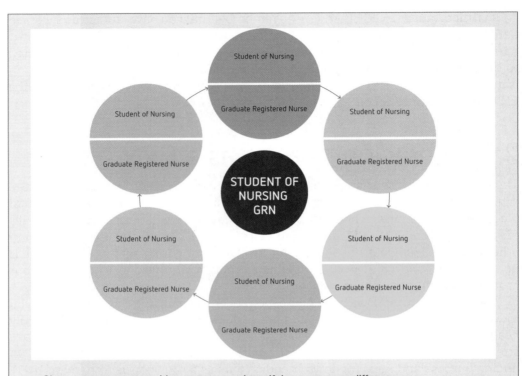

a   Share your responses with your peers and see if there were any differences.
b   Discuss these differences from the perspective of learning and expanding your scope of
     practice and professional development.

HOW DID YOU GO?

Did you see how many skills and how much knowledge you already hold that you will use as a GRN?
As a GRN, you are well prepared for practice, and if you work within your scope of practice and gain
assistance when needed, you will be a safe practitioner. An important aspect of your professional
identity is your ability to provide safe care and to keep yourself safe, which you should be very mindful
of during your transition to practice because a lack of confidence in your ability to practice safely can
easily undermine your sense of self.

2.4 Role stress and the collaborative team

role stress
The level of stress that is
experienced by a person
in their professional role;
often experienced by those
who are new to a role.

Role stress is well described by Sayers (2020), and different types of
role stress, such as role incongruity, role conflict, role ambiguity and
role overload, can lead the GRN to be unsure of the expectations of
their role and can impact negatively on their ability to identify as a
competent RN. This perception of incompetence could lead the GRN

to work outside of their scope of practice to prove their capabilities to themselves and to others. It is very important for you to understand your role in the clinical context. Understand what will be expected of you and ensure that expectations are within your scope of practice. This will shape your professional identity and personal perceptions as one of a competent beginning RN.

Working with the collaborative team in the development of your professional identity

As a GRN, you will find yourself working closely with a collaborative **transdisciplinary** team. The team will vary and be dependent upon the clinical area and the needs of the patients in your care. For example, a community health care team may be quite small and include the community nurse, local pharmacist, physiotherapist and the patient's general practitioner. For a person hospitalised with a complex health condition, the team will expand to include all allied health care professionals, investigative specialists, a large speciality nursing team and medical doctors who work from different speciality areas of practice.

> **transdisciplinary**
> A situation where different health disciplines' borders are blurred or crossed.

Regardless of whether you are working with a small or a large health care team, the health care team is an excellent source of support and guidance for you as a beginner and will provide you with valuable resources to assist you in your professional development (Slusser et al., 2019). It is imperative, however, that they understand your role in the collaborative team. The team members may not have worked with a GRN previously and may expect you to work from the position of an experienced RN. Pointing out that you are in your early years of practice and the clinical environment is unfamiliar to you will give them the opportunity to know how to support you in your practice. Taking on the identity as a member of the collaborative team who is a beginner in the area of practice, means you can gain support from all members of the team and from a multidisciplinary perceptive. It is an excellent opportunity to learn and develop professionally and identify as a competent RN.

PRACTICAL APPLICATION: SEEKING THE BEST SUPPORT FROM WITHIN THE HEALTH CARE TEAM

You are employed as a GRN in your first month of practice working in an orthopaedic unit. You have a supportive collaborative team of health care professionals who you know you can approach at any time for advice and support. You are struggling to make a clinical decision about a patient who has unresolved pain post total knee replacement. You have recognised that your knowledge about this procedure is foundational only and that you have reached the peak of your scope of practice in this area.

> a   Identify three different health care professionals in the orthopaedic collaborative team (this includes another nurse) who you would approach to assist you in your decision making.

> b   Describe the type of questions you would ask and how you could frame them to obtain the support that you need.

> c   Work in a small group and write a script and role-play how you as the GRN would approach each of the health care professionals for advice. This activity should show the different use of language dependent upon the health care professional's speciality area.

HOW DID YOU GO?

There are a number of health care professionals in the team who you could approach for support. The important point is to be very clear as to who will be the 'best' person to ask. Don't always go to the team leader or to the doctor, there may be other more suitable members of the team, such as the pharmacist or the physiotherapist, who can assist you.

2.5 Working from the position of being a lifelong learner

lifelong learner
A person who independently seeks knowledge and information. A perpetual learner.

To identify as a **lifelong learner** is imperative for your professional development and will be a catalyst for you to move towards being an expert RN. **Lifelong learning** is propelled by the expectation of working from a position of curiosity and critical reflection, which is a professional standard of practice for the RN. As a student, you were expected to demonstrate higher-order thinking skills, such as analysis, justification and critical thinking, and you would have been assessed at this level of thinking in the clinical context. As a GRN, the expectation is that you will now independently work from this platform of intrinsic motivation, and as one who is constantly seeking knowledge and understanding.

lifelong learning
Learning that is motivated by an intrinsic desire to gain knowledge for both personal and professional reasons.

resilient approach to practice
Growing and developing from experiences, whether they are perceived as positive or negative.

Embracing the attributes of self-motivation, mindfulness and open-mindedness are essential in developing and becoming an autonomous lifelong learner. This includes learning from all experiences, even those that may not have gone as well as you would have liked and you find difficult to revisit. Taking a **resilient approach to practice** will enable you to treat all experiences as learning opportunities that will propel you forward as a lifelong learner.

A resilient approach to practice for the GRN

Being resilient at this time of identity change is important. The term 'resilience' is used widely across nursing practice and is often linked to being able to work through adversity and come out the other side a wiser and healthier person (Daugherty & Steenbergh, 2020). However, resilience in relation to identity change is one of accepting and immersing yourself in your changing role so that you can expand your scope of practice and develop greater knowledge and skills. Resisting the opportunities around you (e.g. avoiding new skills) will hamper your ability to shift your identify from that of a student to an RN. Ultimately this may slow your transition path and impact on your abilities to work effectively in your health care team and to provide safe patient care.

Personal resilience to protect your work–life balance

As a graduate, you will need to be both personally as well as professionally resilient in your attitudes and behaviours. Your personal identity will change as your career influences your lifestyle. Routines will change and you may now be a shift worker who needs to take on different eating and sleeping patterns, and have to plan out opportunities for gatherings with family and friends, which you never had to do before. Your priorities may change, and so could your friendship groups to include those who you work with as you can debrief with them, rather than with friends who do not understand your situation or where you think you may breach your professional boundaries if you speak of work matters.

Personal resilience as a GRN means not letting your work invade your personal space. As a lifelong learner, you will be revising medical conditions and working

work–life balance
A situation where a person feels that their work life and personal life is at a point where one complements the other.

through study modules as part of your professional development. It is important that you are mindful of the time this takes and be sure to allocate times where you can rest and relax with family and friends. Plan out and use your time wisely, and think of options that will provide you with an effective **work–life balance**.

CASE **STUDY**

WORK–LIFE BALANCE: EXAMPLE

Tom has to complete three nursing modules that are particular to his clinical area. Each module takes about 10 hours to complete. Tom lives with his partner and three young children and when he is home, he prefers to spend his time with them as much as possible. To meet both personal and professional needs, Tom goes to work 1.5 hours earlier on a late shift and stays back 1.5 hours after an early shift to work through the modules. He does this about three times per week. Tom has found that he can concentrate better on the modules in the hospital library and has often found a nurse educator there if he needs assistance. Tom feels that this approach gives him a sense of control over work not invading his home life, and that he can give the modules the time and energy needed to complete them well.

a   What current demands do you have on your time that could be minimised using a creative problem-solving approach?

b   How does the example of Tom demonstrate a resilient approach to professional practice?

HOW DID YOU GO?

Thinking outside of the square and adjusting your usual methods and routines can enable you to approach demands and problems with a fresh and novel approach. Reconsider timeframes, places and people who you could involve to bring about change and improve situations. This form of open-mindedness means that you will approach problems from a resilient and objective problem-solving position.

Professional resilience to enhance your professional growth

Taking a resilient approach to professional practice, by responding positively to change and new learning opportunities, enables you to identify as a beginner who is moving towards becoming an expert nurse. An area of particular concern for graduates, where a resilient approach to practice is needed, is one of engaging with the professional team to enable a shared decision-making approach to practice (Conway, 2021). Graduates have reported feeling as though they should not have a voice as their knowledge and experience is too limited. If you pursue this approach over the long term, then the collaborative team will identify you as someone who is incapable of clinical reasoning and does not have the knowledge or skills to represent the nursing discipline. It is, therefore, essential that you remember your roles and responsibilities as an RN, and advocate for the patient from within your scope of practice. This will take courage and practice, but if you are confident that your position is one of safe practice that it is informed by knowledge and clinical experience, then you can speak with authority and credibility.

Reflecting on all your professional experiences and working as a lifelong learner to move towards expertise is the resilient approach to practice. Reflection can take many forms, with some graduates preferring to journal their experiences, and others preferring to discuss their experiences with a mentor or to debrief with other graduates, preceptors or educators. However you choose to reflect on your clinical experiences, it needs to be done in a safe and positive environment with an objective approach to your thinking and reasoning. Ultimately, you are seeking understanding and knowledge for future practice, rather than looking for someone to blame for a particular outcome.

As a graduate, there may be times when you make clinical judgement errors, forget to complete a task or communicate something with the team. This is part of your journey of learning. The important action is to rectify the situation as quickly as possible, admit your error and work towards addressing the situation. You then identify as an honest and trustworthy health care professional. Your resilience and desire to learn from situations will allow you to analyse and look objectively and critically at the encounter and work from the experience, rather than be embroiled in the experience. Your depth of learning and reasoning will lead you to a greater understanding of how you can work within the health care system to ensure best patient care outcomes.

2.6 Emotional literacy and a resilient approach to practice

The term **emotional literacy** relates to a person's ability to be aware of their own needs and to be able to 'read' the people around them, and is used widely in schools to help children develop an observant approach to life (Waterhouse, 2019). A person's level of emotional literacy informs their **emotional intelligence**, but, more importantly, it is what the GRN does with the information they gain from their emotional literacy that will enable their confidence and resilience to grow in practice (i.e. learning and growing from experiences). If a nurse is blindly unaware of their own needs and their impact on others, then no learning can occur.

emotional literacy
The skill to recognise, express and understand personal responses to situations and also recognising (reading) those of others.

emotional intelligence
The overall ability to gain and apply knowledge and skills in relation to emotions.

For example, a graduate nurse working in a general practice clinic is struggling with a complex dressing. She is being extra careful as it is a slow healing wound, and she wants to be sure that the dressing is effective and won't fall off. By using her emotional literacy, the graduate senses/reads that the patient is becoming frustrated with her slowness. She asks the patient, 'is everything is alright?' The patient states that she is worried she will miss her usual bus. It is with empathy that the GRN can then assist the patient to find transport, and to also understand that she should always check with the patient first regarding their timetable.

This graduate is developing a resilient approach to practice by learning positively from her experiences.

PRACTICAL APPLICATION: RECOGNISING EMOTIONAL LITERACY SKILLS TO DEVELOP RESILIENCE IN PRACTICE

In small groups, describe a situation where you were challenged, and you could have learnt more from the experience but found it difficult to 'unpack'.

Using the characteristics of emotional intelligence as a reference, discuss with your peers how each of the emotional literacy skills listed below could assist you to understand the situation more thoroughly, so as to develop a resilient approach to practice from the experience you described.

	Emotional literacy skills	Inform resilience in practice
Self-awareness	'Was I curious about the experiences?' 'Did I seek feedback from others?' 'Am I aware of my own self-motivation/empowerment?' 'Am I aware of my own self confidence?'	
Social awareness	'Did I demonstrate empathy for others?' 'Was I an approachable and active listener?' 'Was I aware of my influence on others?' 'Did I understand cultural and environmental influences?'	
Self-regulation	'Did I maintain self-control?' 'Did I actively learn from the experience?' 'Did I work from previous feedback?' 'Was I open-minded to positive influences?' 'Was I flexible and adaptable in my response?'	
Social regulation	'Was I an effective communicator?' 'Was I an inspirational leader?' 'Did I use effective mentoring skills?' 'Did I effectively work through any conflict?' 'Did I work collaboratively with others?'	

Source: adapted from Purushothaman, R. (2021). *Emotional intelligence*. Sage Publications.

HOW DID YOU GO?

A resilient approach to practice is an approach that is driven by an honest desire to grow your personal self and professional self. When you worked through the questions above, you may have realised that you didn't pursue some of the emotional literacy elements, such as 'Did I seek feedback from others?' or 'Did I demonstrate empathy for others?'. That is an important realisation as you will then understand how you can learn more from your experiences and become more self-reliant and resilient in your practice approaches.

FOCUS POINTS AND MOVING FORWARD

This chapter focused on the changing identity that you, as a GRN, will experience and assume as your career develops. This can be difficult in the early stages of your transition to practice. It is how you identify yourself that will determine the confidence in which you will express your scope of practice and how you will recognise and move towards opportunities for professional development. Adapting a resilient approach to practice will enable you to learn from experiences, and it will assist you in understanding how your changed roles and responsibilities enable you to become the RN that you want to become.

DISCUSSION POINTS

1. It is important that a person's professional identity does not overwhelm or subsume their personal identity. Discuss.

_____

_____

_____

_____

2. Discuss the value of the collaborative team supporting the GRN in their goal to being a lifelong learner.

_____

_____

_____

_____

3. Taking a resilient approach to practice is essential for the GRN to learn from experiences. Discuss how this occurs.

_____

_____

_____

_____

REFERENCES

Alexander, S., & Stewart, L. (2020). Establishing and maintaining a professional identity: Portfolios and career progression. In E. Chang & J. Daly (Eds.), _Transitions in nursing. Preparing for professional practice_ (5th ed., ch 17). Elsevier.

Black, B. (2019). _Professional nursing: Concepts and challenges_ (9th ed.). Elsevier.

Conway, J. (2021). Connecting clinical and theoretical knowledge for practice. In D. Daly & D. Jackson (Eds.), _Contexts of nursing_ (6th ed., ch 20). Elsevier.

Daugherty, D., & Steenbergh, T. (2020). A rose by any other name: a common language. In A. Baldwin, B. Bunting, D. Daugherty, L. Lewis & T. Steenbergh (Eds.), _Promoting belonging, growth mindset, and resilience to foster student success_ (pp. 11–29). University of South Carolina, National Resource Center for The First-Year Experience and Students in Transition.

Gulliya, T. (2012). _A pilot study testing the effect of the Johari Window on the self-awareness domain of Emotional Intelligence in Generation Y_. Dissertation.

Khan, M. (2021). Imposter syndrome – a particular problem for medical students. _BMJ_, 375, 3048. https://doi.org/10.1136/bmj.n3048

Purushothaman, R. (2021). _Emotional intelligence_. Sage Publications.

Sayers, J. (2020). Preparing for role transition. In E. Chang & J. Daly (Eds.), _Transitions in nursing. Preparing for professional practice_ (5th ed., ch 6). Elsevier.

Slusser, M., Garcia, L., Reed, C-R., & McGinnis, P. (2019). _Foundations of interprofessional collaborative practice in health care_. Elsevier.

Verklan, M. (2007). Johari Window: A model for communicating to each other. _The Journal of Perinatal and Neonatal Nursing, 2192_, 173–174. DOI 10.1097/01.JPN.0000270636.34982.c8

Waterhouse, S. K. (2019). _Emotional literacy: Supporting emotional health and wellbeing in schools_. Routledge.

USEFUL WEBSITES

Nursing and Midwifery Board of Australia, Registered nurse standards for practice, https://www.nursingmidwiferyboard.gov.au/Codes-Guidelines-Statements/Professional-standards/registered-nurse-standards-for-practice.aspx

3 EMBRACING THE ROLES AND RESPONSIBILITIES OF BEING A BEGINNER RN

Learning objectives

Working through this chapter will enable you to:

1. value the professional standards that influence your changing roles and responsibilities as a graduate registered nurse
2. communicate with accuracy and confidence your scope of practice when working independently as a registered nurse
3. embrace the nurse's roles and responsibilities that empower a person to identify and advocate for their rights to express their own health care needs.

Introduction

The health care system is an ever-changing dynamic that is shaped by many factors that both transform and drive health care. As a student you worked within a relatively rigid structure of learning under supervision, but as a graduate registered nurse (GRN) your learning opportunities will be influenced by many other factors. Foremost your learning will be underpinned by your job description, your ability and motivation to learn, the health care team supporting you and the needs of the people in your care. Other platforms, such as digital health mediums and global health initiatives, will also influence your expanding roles and responsibilities as a registered nurse (RN). And, as your experience and knowledge increases, so too will your roles and responsibilities, and you will find your scope of practice expanding every day to accommodate these professional expectations.

3.1 Understanding roles and responsibilities as an RN

Due to the very diverse opportunities for employment in nursing, the 'role' of the RN may vary greatly and will be dependent upon the terms of employment. This may include the context of care (i.e. where you are employed and by whom), the expectations of your role (e.g. clinical or educational), and your level of knowledge and experience (i.e. scope of practice). For example, a nurse's role may be as a clinician, a preceptor, a researcher or a manager. The RN's role is described in the job description and should be carefully reclarified if the nurse achieves promotion or they are seconded or relocated to a different area of practice. As a beginner, your role will include descriptors such as 'expected to independently (and interdependently) provide nursing services in an acute care setting', or 'will work directly with other health care professionals and will report directly to the Nurse Unit Manager'.

The responsibilities that accompany the role for an RN are those tasks or expectations that must be undertaken for the nurse to fulfill the role. Given the breadth of nursing roles, the responsibilities can be quite different for each. In Table 3.1, for example, the responsibilities that accompany a nurse clinicians' role will include the expectations to ensure person-centred care in their practice, maintain safe practices when administering medication or dressing a wound, and work within their scope of practice. These are legal, moral and ethical expectations which are stipulated by the nursing regulatory body (i.e. the Nursing and Midwifery Board of Australia [NMBA]) and by law.

If this concerns you, remember that the Bachelor of Nursing program has provided you with learning opportunities that have prepared you for your roles and responsibilities when working as a GRN. While the Registered nurse standards for practice were primarily put in place to protect and reassure the public of the care that they should expect, the standards and policies are also there to guide you in your practice. If you ensure that you practice your roles and responsibilities within the regulation standards and policies and you work to your scope of practice, be reassured that you are working safely.

▶ Table 3.1 Nurse roles and associated responsibilities

Roles	Responsibilities
Nurse ward clinician	Ensure all care is person-centered Use a collaborative approach to clinical decision making Maintain a safe working environment
Operating theatre nurse	Visit and assess patients prior to surgery Ensure all materials are available for the procedure Meet operating theatre sterility and cleanliness mandates
Primary health care nurse	Assess the social determinants of health that may impact on a person's health Provide primary health promotion support and education Run and manage immunisation clinics
Nurse educator	Design teaching programs that align with the curriculum Assess students based on the stipulated learning outcomes Provide constructive feedback that is student-centered
Nurse administrators	Interview and employ staff to ensure a suitable skill mix Attend to shift rostering that enables staff to be well rested Attend organisational meetings to keep in line with changes and updates

Scope of practice: a nursing responsibility

'Scope of practice' is a term that is used widely in nursing, and it is a responsibility of care that all RNs will practice safely within their scope of practice (NMBA, 2020). It is therefore essential that you can identify what knowledge, competencies and clinical skills you hold at any given time that enable you to provide safe patient care. If you believe that you do not have the knowledge and clinical skills to make a clinical decision or to plan and implement care safely for a patient, then it is outside of your scope of practice. Seeking suitable assistance when care falls outside of your skills and knowledge range is also your responsibility. This enables two positive outcomes. First, the patient receives the health care that they need and, second, you are on the path to expanding your own scope of practice.

Safe patient care is always paramount in your nursing practice, and you will find this is a constant in all policies of practice. This expectation is to not only ensure that the people you care for receive the best evidenced-based care, but also protect yourself from any repercussions of not providing safe practice. As a GRN, there may be occasions where you overlook a patient sign, do not pick up on an omission of care or find that you either miss providing an ordered treatment or have given incorrect treatment. The ramifications of these errors can range from a delay in care, which is easily rectified, to a significant outcome, such as rescheduled surgery or hypoglycaemic events due to inaccurate insulin infusion rates. Even when errors occur, your goal is for safe practice, so you must report the error to your relevant supervisor as soon as you realise the situation. This ensures that the least harm is caused and you are working within the expectations of being an RN.

In the early stages of your transition to practice, when your scope of practice is quite narrow compared to experienced RNs, you may feel as though you are constantly needing assistance and guidance. Remember, you have entered the RN role with a beginning level of knowledge and clinical skills, and that it is very normal for you to need high levels of support at this stage in your career. The breadth and diversity of support is limited only to the support services around you and your ability to seek this out. Certainly, your collaborative health care team is one network that is invaluable to the beginning GRN. Complete the following practical activity so that you have thought about how to gain support from your collaborative team as a GRN.

PRACTICAL APPLICATION: RECOGNISING YOUR SCOPE OF PRACTICE

In groups, discuss and list three unique responsibilities that you think will accompany each of the different nurse roles listed in the table below. Consider if these responsibilities are in your current scope of practice. If not, note what you will need to do to expand your scope of practice so that you can fulfill these responsibilities.

GRN roles	GRN responsibilities	Scope of practice
Day surgery nurse		
Emergency department nurse		
Aged care nurse		
School nurse		
Hospital in the Home nurse		
Post-op recovery nurse		

HOW DID YOU GO?

This exercise provides you with the opportunity to be prepared for when tasks, skills or knowledge requirements are outside of your scope of practice. For example, inserting a nasogastric tube or an indwelling urinary catheter may be something that you have not had the opportunity to practice in the clinical area before. Or you may be unsure of the post-operative care of a patient who has had spinal surgery. Having strategies ready for you to seek advice and support is important in your preparation for practice as a GRN.

3.2 Being an autonomous and independent practitioner

RNs are expected to work autonomously and independently. Working autonomously means that you are working as a professional, making clinical decisions independently within the parameters set by your discipline's regulatory body (Hodge & Varndell, 2018). This includes working independently within your scope of practice and seeking advice when care demands are outside of your scope of practice. It does not mean that you know how to do everything and can't access and utilise the support around you. As a GRN, no one will expect you to be a nursing expert; what they will expect is that you will practice within your scope of practice, you will ask for advice when needed and you will work with the health care team to enable best patient care.

Responsibility and accountability

The responsibilities and accountabilities that accompany independent practice are one of the areas of greatest concern identified by GRNs. As a GRN, you have a responsibility, or a duty of care, to provide the best possible evidence-based, person-centred care for the patient. And while you have always been responsible for the care you provided as a student, the overall responsibility was generally to that of your buddy nurse as well as to the people you were caring for, the health care facility and the university. As a GRN, while you have less people and organisations to be responsible to, your responsibility to these stakeholders is more autonomous. Therefore, if you have any concerns or points to clarify, it is important that you refer to documents such as the International Council of Nurses' Code of Ethics for nurses (ICN, 2021) which explains the professional roles and responsibilities of your new position in the health care system.

Accountability, on the other hand, is where the RN must be able to explain why they chose the care that was provided and be answerable to the health care outcomes. This includes being able to explain clinical reasoning decisions from when the patient is first assessed to the evaluation and reflection of the care, the RN's communication practices and their ability to work within their scope of practice (Hodge & Varndell, 2018). The NMBA's clinical Decision-making framework explains how accountability is an important aspect of independent practice for the RN. Not only is it a regulatory expectation, but being accountable is reassuring for the patients in your care as your commitment to accepting care outcomes reassures them that you are a professional who takes their role and responsibilities seriously (Yuan & Murphy, 2019).

While there is an increase in both responsibility and accountability for the GRN from being more independent in their practice and being answerable to outcomes, the changes are probably not quite as significant as you may think, and you will never be alone when making decisions if you need support.

Delegation of care

Delegation of care is a response to the number of unregulated and less qualified nurses working in the health care sector who need support and supervision when providing some patient care needs. The Nursing and Midwifery Board of Australia defines delegation as 'the relationship that exists when one member of the multidisciplinary healthcare team delegates aspects of care, which they are competent to perform and which they would normally perform themselves, to another health professional or health care worker' (NMBA, 2020, p. 12). Even as a beginner, you will be expected to delegate care, but due to your developing scope of practice, you may also be delegated a care task.

Being fully cognisant of your own scope of practice is the first essential step in determining delegation of care. This is essential for when you need to provide supervisory support when delegating care or accepting a task delegated to you.

Delegation is an RN role that is complex and requires an approach to practice that is patient-centred and collaborative (Walker et al., 2021). Ultimately, the RN has a responsibility to ensure that all patients receive the care they need and if that care is not provided, then the RN is accountable and must answer for the omissions. Knowing how to delegate and accept delegation safely and effectively is a role that you are responsible for from the first day of practice as an RN. While you may not have had a lot of experience in this area of practice as a student, you will find that you will develop these skills quickly and effectively.

PRACTICAL APPLICATION: THE PROCESS OF DELEGATION

To work as an Australian RN, you must understand the NMBA's process of delegation. Use the following table as a guide to assist you in your understanding of the process.

a   List the four phases of delegation as described in the NMBA's Decision-making framework (pp. 9–10).

b   Write a summary of key factors to describe the purpose of each of the phases.

c   Discuss the scenario where you are a GRN (day 5 as a graduate), and you are to delegate care for a patient who needs to have a medicated moisturising cream applied to his arms and legs.

d   Working through the four phases of delegation, describe the procedure to ensure that care is provided safely in the above scenario.

Phases of delegation	Summary of key factors	Scope of practice
Phase 1		
Phase 2		
Phase 3		
Phase 4		

HOW DID YOU GO?

Delegation is a skill that you need to learn quickly as a GRN. You will have staff looking to be delegated tasks and who will want to work within their scope of practice. Delegation is important because as a beginner some aspects of RN care will be outside your scope of practice and you will need to gain support from others to learn the skill yourself. Take your time to expand your scope of practice so that your delegation of tasks expands as well. Remember, though, that there are care needs that can always be delegated to others to enable you to work on developing your own scope of practice.

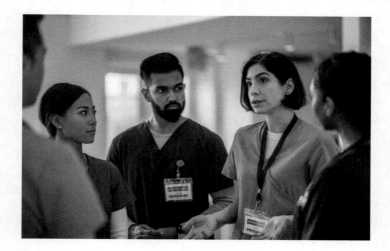

Source: iStock.com/FatCamera

Delegation of care means that everyone's needs are met. This includes the people in your care as well as members of the health care team.

3.3 Advocacy

The role of **advocate** is central to that of being an RN (Kalaitzidis & Jewell, 2020). There are many forms of advocacy, with delegation itself being one form. The term 'health advocacy' is explained in the NMBA's Code of conduct, and describes the role of the nurse as an advocate who ensures that there is health care equity, where all persons receive access to health care from the position of justice and fairness. This includes those groups where there are noted disparities in health care provision, such as people with disabilities, refugees and Aboriginal and Torres Strait Islander peoples. If, as a beginner, you find advocacy expectations to be concerning and outside your scope of practice, then thinking about supporting vulnerable populations from the perspective of the Australian Charter of Healthcare Rights may be a more structured

advocate
Someone who recognises and supports others.

approach for you. Either way, ensuring that health care is available to all persons in an equitable manner is an essential point of advocacy in nursing practice.

Patient advocacy

Patient advocacy has been embraced as part of the nurse's role to ensure the patient's position and concerns are heard and understood. Patient advocacy has been described as 'speaking for the person'; however, our role is to support people to speak for themselves and to **empower** them so their own voices are heard (Butts & Rich, 2018). If we 'speak for the person' then we take away their independence and their confidence as a person who can self-manage their own care. It is also important to realise that being a patient advocate is not a 'nursing only' role – all health care workers have a role and a responsibility to advocate for the people in their care. Advocacy extends to the collaborative team in that all members of the team, including the GRN, will advocate for the patient from the perspective of their discipline and will work collaboratively to ensure holistic patient-centered care is achieved.

empower
To encourage a person to feel more confident and able to achieve a desired outcome.

Workplace advocacy

While patient advocacy is generally considered to be a direct approach to support a patient's needs, it is equally important that the workplace environment in which care is provided is safe and that the health care professionals themselves have the capability to provide safe care. *Workplace advocacy* considers the context of care or the environment in which care is undertaken, and all other aspects of the workplace. It may also include the workforce, but this is discussed separately. As a GRN, you have a responsibility to ensure that the workplace is a safe place to practice and it may include aspects such as ensuring floors are not slippery from spilled water, that correct medication checks and policies are followed, and that faulty equipment is reported and replaced. There is no excuse for not advocating for a safe workplace and you will be held accountable if an injury occurs because of your lack of action to address a workplace issue.

Workforce advocacy is also an important aspect of safe patient care, and while as a GRN you will not be in charge of rostering, employing staff, formally mentoring or seeking replacement staff, you do have a responsibility to be aware of and report workforce issues that may impact on safe patient care. As a GRN, it is imperative that you have the support that you need to be able to work safely and effectively. If, for example, you note that the team does not have the skill mix to provide the support you will need during the shift, then you need to report this to your supervisor and negotiate the support that you need. You also have a responsibility to ensure that all team members work to their scope of practice. This occurs by delegating tasks to those who will be able to meet the needs of the patients in your care.

There is also an expectation that you will speak out if a member of the workforce is not able to provide safe care. Mandatory reporting processes are in place so that all health care professionals can identify when it is reasonably believed that a member of the workforce is not meeting the expected standards of practice. The mandatory notification guidelines (Australian Health Practitioner Regulation Agency, 2020) give very specific examples and expectations and if a health care practitioner is not performing to their discipline's standards of practice, supervisors need to be notified. Circumstances stated in the guidelines include issues due to a physical or mental impairment, intoxication while practicing, a significant departure from accepted professional standards or sexual misconduct. As a GRN, you would advocate for patients' safety and report your concerns to your preceptor or team leader.

Table 3.2 lists some suggested advocacy responsibilities for GRNs.

▶ **Table 3.2** Suggested advocacy responsibilities for the GRN

Patient	Workplace	Workforce
Uphold Australian Charter of Healthcare Rights (ACSQHC) • Access • Safety • Respect • Partnership • Information • Privacy • Give feedback	• Ensure environment is safe • Safe equipment • Policies and guidelines available • Evidence-based practice supported • Functioning computer-based systems • Organisational supports in place (places for staff to take their breaks / functioning bathrooms)	• Skill mix can meet the needs of the people being cared for • Roster system allows for rest and recovery • Staff are given the opportunity for professional development • Workloads allow for best practice

PRACTICAL APPLICATION: ADVOCACY

You are working in a busy surgical ward. It is your first night shift and your allocated preceptor has called in sick. When you observe the nursing team on the night shift, there are only two RNs, one is team leader and the other is a graduate with only three months more experience than yourself. The remainder of the staff are enrolled nurses. Your patient allocation has responsibilities that are outside of your scope of practice. You are aware that you are going to need to speak up so that you can have the workforce support you will need for the shift.

Discuss in small groups how you will:
• advocate for yourself so that you have the adequate support to care for the patients you have been allocated
• approach the team leader at the beginning of the shift to highlight the areas where you will need support
• be sure that the team leader has provided you with a response that provides the support that you will need
• create a clear plan of where and when you will need support and be sure that this is booked in.

HOW DID YOU GO?

As a GRN, it is vital that you can express your needs so that you can gain the required support. You need to consider your scope of practice, the allocated work and the team around you. Plan out your support early in the shift and set up key timeframes and availability windows. Reassess your needs as the shift progresses and reset your supports as changes occur.

FOCUS POINTS AND MOVING FORWARD

There is great anticipation around the shift from student to RN and the changing roles and responsibilities of the new position. While it should not be taken lightly, your preparation for practice has taken you a long way towards preparing for these changes. Being responsible and accountable are expectations that reflect your ability to practice professionally and safely. When you understand your scope of practice and work from a clinical reasoning position, you will not only provide safe care to your patients but you will be safe as well.

DISCUSSION POINTS

1. Think about the area of practice you would prefer to work in as a GRN, and discuss the roles that are of most interest to you and why this is so.

   _____

   _____

   _____

   _____

2. Discuss how you will be able to work more independently in your role as an RN when delegating care to others.

   _____

   _____

   _____

   _____

3. Discuss how the Australian Charter of Healthcare Rights could assist you to recognise situations where you would need to advocate for the person in your care.

_____

_____

_____

_____

REFERENCES

Australian Health Practitioner Regulation Agency. (2020). _Mandatory notifications: What you need to know._ https://www.medicalboard.gov.au/sitecore/content/Home/Notifications/mandatorynotifications.aspx

Butts, J., & Rich, K. (2018). Ethics in professional nursing practice. In K. Masters (Ed.). _Role development in professional nursing practice_ (pp. 563–638). Jones and Bartlett Learning.

Hodge, A. & Varndell, W. (2018). _Professional transitions in nursing. A guide to practice in the Australian healthcare system_. Allen and Unwin.

International Council of Nurses. (2021). _ICN Code of Ethics for Nurses_. https://www.icn.ch/system/files/2021-10/ICN_Code-of-Ethics_EN_Web_0.pdf

Kalaitzidis, E., & Jewell, P. (2020). The concept of advocacy in nursing. A critical analysis. _The Health Care Manager, 39_(2), 77–84. https://doi.org/10.1097/HCM.0000000000000079

Nursing and Midwifery Board of Australia. (2020). Decision-making framework for nursing and midwifery. https://www.nursingmidwiferyboard.gov.au/codes-guidelines-statements/frameworks.aspx

Walker, F., Ball, M., Cleary, S., & Pisani, H. (2021). Transparent teamwork: The practice of supervision and delegation within the multi-tiered nursing team. _Nursing Inquiry, 28_(4), e12413. https://doi.org/10.1111/nin.12413

Yuan, S., & Murphy, J. (2019). _Partnerships in nursing care: A concept analysis_. TMR Publishing Group.

USEFUL WEBSITES

Australian Charter of Healthcare Rights, ACSQHC, https://www.safetyandquality.gov.au/consumers/working-your-healthcare-provider/australian-charter-healthcare-rights

International Council of Nurses (ICN), ICN Code of Ethics for Nurses, https://www.icn.ch/system/files/2021-10/ICN_Code-of-Ethics_EN_Web_0.pdf

Nursing and Midwifery Board of Australia, Code of conduct for nurses, https://www.nursingmidwiferyboard.gov.au/codes-guidelines-statements/professional-standards.aspx

Nursing and Midwifery Board of Australia, Decision-making framework for nursing and midwifery, https://www.nursingmidwiferyboard.gov.au/codes-guidelines-statements/frameworks.aspx

Nursing and Midwifery Board of Australia, Registered nurse standards for practice, https://www.nursingmidwiferyboard.gov.au/Codes-Guidelines-Statements/Professional-standards/registered-nurse-standards-for-practice.aspx

PART 2

PREPARING FOR THE HEALTH CARE ENVIRONMENT

Learning outcomes

1. Describe the different health care environments in which you may find employment as a graduate registered nurse.
2. Anticipate health care changes that will impact on you as a health care professional when working in the developing health care system in Australia.
3. Plan and articulate the changes that will occur as a result of your transition to practice as a graduate registered nurse.

Preamble

Health care environments vary as much as the people who seek health care. One significant advantage of selecting a career as a registered nurse (RN) is the almost infinite number of choices as to where and how you may practice your discipline. These opportunities are enhanced by the breadth of knowledge and skills that come your way, expand your scope of practice and add to your job satisfaction. And it is not only the clinical service that is varied, the geographical place of practice and the health care team who you work with can also be very diverse. It is this diverse collective of nursing practice opportunities that enables the RN to regroup and retrain into different areas of the health care system. It is important, therefore, that as a graduate RN (GRN) you don't limit your ambitions and career goals to one area of practice as there is always the potential for adventure and change into a new avenue of health care.

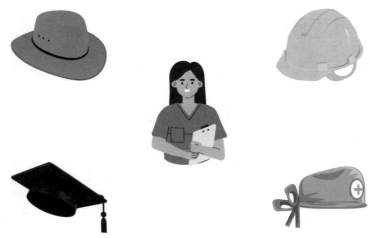

Sources (from left to right): Shutterstock.com/sreville; Shutterstock.com/tatianakabakova; Shutterstock.com/GoodStudio; Shutterstock.com/koya979; Shutterstock.com/johavel

4

PREPARING FOR A NEW HEALTH CARE ENVIRONMENT AS A GRN

Learning objectives

Working through this chapter will enable you to:

1. value the population trends that influence nursing employment opportunities in Australia
2. compare opportunities in different health care environments
3. incorporate health promotion and disease prevention into professional practice
4. visualise nursing opportunities within different contexts of care
5. understand how the National Health Priority Areas will be fundamental in your preparation for practice.

Introduction

The mantra 'wherever there are people, there are nurses' provides you with a sense of the breadth of nursing-related positions available and offers you a starting point for where you may look for employment as a graduate registered nurse (GRN). Nursing has always provided a diversity of practice opportunities that also allow travel and flexibility around family commitments and postgraduate studies. You may think that planning your nursing career while a GRN is too early, but your career goals will take you to a place where you will celebrate your achievements, and it is your professional vision that guides your career journey. It is never too early to start thinking about your career and the environment in which you would like to live and work. Websites such as the Australian College of Nursing Career Hub are good starting points to help you think about your preferences and how you plan to get to there.

4.1 Geographical location

The geographic location of the health care facility, the health care services that are offered and the people who you are providing health care to are influencing factors as to where you will find employment. One of the health care challenges for Australians is that Australia is a large country with a relatively small population, most of whom are settled on the eastern seaboard. Australia's different geographical areas are categorised in different ways. One method is to consider the 'Remoteness Areas of Australia' (Bishop et al., 2017). These tools of measurement show the distance between inhabited places. Other maps show the sparsity of the population per square kilometre. Australia has an average of 3.3 people per square kilometre; however, as is demonstrated in the map in Figure 4.1, metropolitan areas see a population of >100 people per square kilometre, but in the most **remote** areas <0.1 person per square kilometre.

remote
In this context, the measurement and extent of distance and space in Australia.

acute care
Care of health problems that are short lived.

The spread of the population in a country can influence where you will find a nursing position. This does not mean that there are no nursing roles in rural and remote areas of Australia, or that the positions in larger centres are only focused on **acute care** needs of people (see also Figure 4.2). What is important to remember is that nurses are involved at all levels of health care, and when thinking about an area of practice that may be of interest to you, think about your experiences as a student in the clinical area as a starting point only and do not limit yourself to mainstream health care hospitals and facilities.

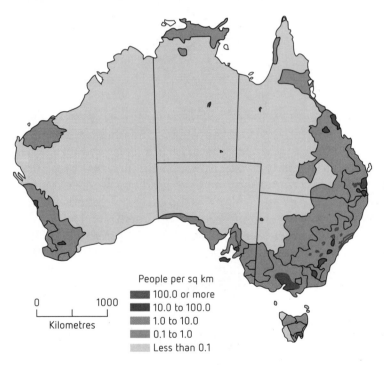

People per sq km
- 100.0 or more
- 10.0 to 100.0
- 1.0 to 10.0
- 0.1 to 1.0
- Less than 0.1

0   1000

Kilometres

Source: Australian Bureau of Statistics

▶ **Figure 4.1** Population density, Australia – June 2018

Health services across the country

The distance between health care services propelled Australia to engage in telehealth in the last century with telegrams, two-way radios and telephones being the initial mediums for communication. With communication capability expanding to internet connections and there are more sophisticated tools in the form of high-tech cameras and information sharing systems, health care professionals around the country can now diagnose and treat conditions for people who would have needed to travel long distances and wait lengthy periods of time for support. So too has health care travel safety improved, with outfitted transport vehicles that can move patients between centres safely in the hands of dedicated health care teams. Joining nursing special interest groups is a good way to start looking for employment and networking with people who may work in the areas that interest you. The Australian College of Nursing provides the Nursing Now website, which clearly describes the global changes in nursing and how you can be a part of them.

4.2 Working within different health care environments

The diversity of health care sectors where you can find employment is just one of the reasons why nursing is such a valuable occupation. Deciding where your preferences lie may take some time, but understanding the fundamental areas of practice is a good starting point. Health care is often divided into broad streams such as acute care, **chronic care** and primary care (see Figure 4.2). It is important to realise that these streams of care are provided across the lifespan and can be needed by any age group of people. Often the mindset is that only older people have chronic conditions and need palliative care. But this is incorrect as a child may need chronic care support with a medical diagnosis of cystic fibrosis or an older adult may need acute care support with a diagnosis of appendicitis (Edelman & Kudzma, 2018). The thought that only older people need rehabilitation support or end of life care is a misnomer as all people need health care support at all levels of care at any age or stage of their life.

chronic care
Long-term care of health problems that are ongoing.

To clarify, acute care is provided in typically curative situations, such as for injuries, diseases, investigations and surgeries, that require a short timeframe of treatment and recovery. Chronic care, on the other hand, is for when the person has a medical condition or injury that is long lasting. This may include autoimmune disorders, such as diabetes, or degenerative disorders, such as motor neurone disease. There are also non-communicable diseases and communicable diseases, such as cardiovascular disease and malaria, that create long-term health difficulties. These conditions ultimately require nurses who are specialised in rehabilitative care,

ACUTE CARE NURSING	CHRONIC CARE NURSING	PRIMARY HEALTH CARE NURSING
Neurological	Hospital in the Home	General practice clinics
Surgical/operating theatre	Community health nurse	School nurse
Intensive care	Acute care wards; e.g. vascular	Occupational health and safety
Emergency department	Rehabilitation wards; e.g. spinal injury	Child health clinics
Geriatric acute care	Oncology/endocrine/respiratory	Correctional health nursing
Day surgery	Aged care: independent living/dementia care	Refugee health care
Outpatients	Palliative care	Drug and alcohol support

▶ Figure 4.2 Examples of types of health care

self-care
A focus on your own needs to ensure best health outcomes.

palliative care and end of life care. While **self-care** is identified as the forerunner in independent health care, health promotion and disease prevention are typically delineated into three different levels of care and are discussed in the next section.

4.3 Health promotion and disease prevention health care

primary prevention
Proactive interventions to prevent disease or illness.

secondary prevention
Identifying a disease or condition in its early stages to prevent progression.

tertiary prevention
Preventing the escalation of an existing disease or condition.

self-manage
When a person can independently manage their ill health.

The first level or **primary prevention** (pre-diagnosis) is where screening for a disease or condition is the aim. The person is generally symptom free. **Secondary prevention** (early diagnosis) is to identify a health problem early, where treatments can be less complex and curative. **Tertiary prevention** strategies are implemented when the person has been diagnosed with a chronic condition and care is in place to ensure quality of life (Naidoo & Wills, 2016). All aim for the patient to ultimately **self-manage** and maintain their own health and wellbeing to the highest possible level. This will not only give the person a sense of control and wellbeing but will also reduce the burden of the disease that chronic conditions can place on the health care system.

An important point to make here is that health promotion is not only a role for nurses working in the community. Health promotion on all levels occurs within the hospital environment and some people may need all levels of prevention support to achieve health and wellbeing (Tveiten, 2021). Working with people who have complex health care needs takes skill and experience to be able to address all their health promotion needs (see Figure 4.3).

CASE **STUDY**

HEALTH PROMOTION – EXAMPLE

An obese man, Jason, who is a long-term tobacco smoker with chronic asthma is admitted to the medical ward as he has a chest infection and is ordered intravenous antibiotic treatment. During the admission, Jason tells you that he does not wear his seatbelt when driving his car as he finds it too uncomfortable due to his current size. Thinking about this case study scenario, it is clear that Jason needs primary prevention support to wear his seat belt when driving in the car, secondary prevention support to address his obesity and tobacco use and tertiary prevention support to address his chronic asthma.

a   In small groups, discuss the difference between the three levels of health promotion that Jason requires.

b   Discuss why all three levels of health promotion should be implemented with a person with a chronic condition.

c   How would you prioritise and plan the care for Jason?

HOW DID YOU GO?

Being able to identify the three levels of health promotion is important for Jason to know how to self-care and to be aware of which levels are preventative, curative or are long-term conditions. As a nurse, it is important to not 'give up' on a patient because of their chronic condition. Implementing all levels of health promotion ensures that the patient achieves their highest quality of health and life.

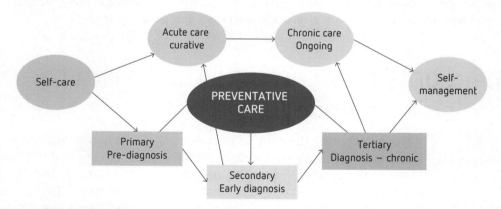

▸ Figure 4.3 Types of health promotion and disease prevention

Due to the increasing rates of non-communicable chronic diseases, you will find that many people you care for will have an underlying chronic illness that has either been exacerbated by an acute illness or has deteriorated. When it is stated that people are getting sicker, it is often referring to the underlying comorbidities that already place the person in a vulnerable position. To understand more about the health care needs of the Australian population and the current plans put in place by the Australian Government to address these needs, refer to the National Strategic

Framework for Chronic Conditions (see the list of useful websites at the end of the chapter). This will help you understand the importance of a dedicated workforce and where job opportunities may be of interest to you.

REFLECTION: FINDING YOUR PROFESSIONAL FOOTPRINT

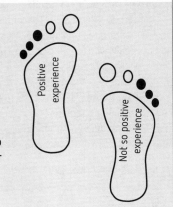

a   Think about an area of nursing practice that you particularly enjoyed during your placement.
b   Now think about one that you did not find so engaging or rewarding.
c   Discuss this with members of your class, then list what influenced your thinking for both areas. Was it the nursing care that you provided or the staff you worked with, or was there a more deep-seated reason behind your response?
    Being aware of what is influencing your choices will help you to make informed choices that may have lifelong implications for your career choice and progression.

HOW DID YOU GO?

Were you able to identify the factors that influenced your response to the clinical experience? Being aware of the situation around you and how you respond to it allows you to understand the impact that your experiences may have on your professional footprint and your professional identity.

4.4 Context of care and the health care environment

context of care
The place where care is provided.

When considering the **context of care** it should be noted that it is not static and will change depending upon the place of care and the care needs of the person (Kearney-Nunnery, 2020). For example, dressing a wound in a person's home will demand a different approach to practice than if the procedure was undertaken in a hospital environment. While the wound care remains the same, how the nurse approaches the care, remembering that they are working in someone's home, requires a very different approach to practice. Hence the environment influences the context of care.

Broadly, health care is provided at primary, secondary, tertiary and quandary levels of care. These levels of care influence the health care services that are available to people and therefore influences the types of available services that the nurse may work within. As you think about where you may prefer to practice as an RN, it is important for you to understand each area and how it will shape your role if working within that environment.

Levels of health care services

The different levels of care are another conduit for nurse employment with both geographical and clinical conditions influencing practice opportunities. As mentioned, they are referred to in the Australian health system as **primary**, **secondary**, **tertiary** and **quandary** levels of care (see Table 4.1).

Primary services are the first point of contact where patient's health care needs are assessed and managed, or they may be referred for further investigations to specialist health care professionals. Nurses often work in primary health care environments in the roles of general practice nurses, community health nurses or school nurses. Small rural hospitals will be supported by general practitioners (GPs) or a medical superintendent at a primary service level, and nursing care is general by nature. Patients with complex care needs that cannot be addressed will be transferred to a larger and more resourced centre. As a GRN, working in primary services is an excellent way to understand health care from the perspective of the first contact point, where patients are initially seeking assistance, or from a primary health screening point where support in the form of healthy lifestyle choices can be supported.

Secondary services are those where specialist medical doctors and more advanced medical imaging and pathology services are available in both a private and public hospital domain. Specialist doctors are those such as paediatricians, general surgeons and obstetricians, and may include GPs who specialise in particular areas; for example, women's health. Specialised community health care teams and rehabilitation services are available and include all levels of allied health care professionals. Nurses are an important part of these collaborative teams and may work as practice nurses in specialised doctor's rooms. Nurses also make up a large proportion of the health care team at secondary care hospital wards, which are more specialised and involve both acute and chronic care needs. As a GRN, you will find graduate positions are often available in these health care areas and it is here that the student and graduate nurse is first introduced to speciality areas of practice.

Tertiary services are regarded as the highest level of health care, where care is provided to patients who are very sick and with complex needs and are generally only available in large metropolitan centres of practice. The highest level of medical imaging and pathology diagnostics occurs within these health care environments, with hospitals providing highly specialised care in specific areas of practice. Sub-speciality doctors, such as orthopaedic surgeons who specialise in knee replacements or endocrinologists who only work in the area of cystic fibrosis, pave the way for RNs to take on a more specialised area of practice.

Quandary level of care is when very highly specialised and unique services are provided. It is usually only a small number of tertiary hospitals that provide these services; for example, organ transplant services. Nurses who work in these areas of practice are usually experienced with postgraduate qualifications in their practice area.

primary level of care
The first point of contact with a health care professional.

secondary level of care
Care that includes specialist medical doctors and more advanced medical imaging and pathology services in both a private and public hospital domain.

tertiary level of care
Includes the highest-level medical, nursing and allied health specialist care and high-end investigative procedures and treatments.

quandary level of care
Unique, highly specialised care facilities, such as transplant services.

▶ Table 4.1 Levels of health care

Level	Health care service	Nurse's role
Primary	Clinic, GP practice Small hospital or community centre Aged care services	Broad scope of practice Across the lifespan
Secondary	Specialised doctors, pathology and biomedical services Hospital wards – unique to patients' needs	Specialised scope of practice Focused care on age groups and medical conditions
Tertiary	Highly specialised doctors and investigative services More complex and life-threatening care services Hospital wards – unique to medical conditions or severity of care needed	May be specialised or highly specialised nursing care and scope of practice Increasing complexity demanding postgraduate education
Quandary	Highest specialty area Unique to some tertiary hospitals	Highest specialty care scope of practice

Across all of these levels of health care, the context of care will differ and this will influence the roles and responsibilities that you will accept as an RN. The context influences how you will care for the person, who will need to be involved in the care and what processes will need to be put in place. Complete the following practical activity to see if you can identify the differences in nursing care that will be needed dependent upon the care environment.

PRACTICAL APPLICATION: WORKING WITHIN DIFFERENT CONTEXTS OF CARE – A COMPARISON

A 3-year-old child spills a saucepan of hot water onto themselves and experiences full thickness burns to their torso. In this activity, there are two different care environments for you to consider. Review the nursing responsibilities carefully. Remember that in a rural setting you are the first responder, whereas in the tertiary care unit, the family has had support from others before they arrive in the ward. Think about which area you would prefer to be involved in.

Paediatric tertiary hospital burns unit RN responsibilities	Primary rural emergency department RN responsibilities
Transferred to the ward directly from emergency department. **Nurses' role on admission:** Maintain fluid balance Pain relief Wound care Prepare for operating theatre for debridement of wounds or skin grafts to wounds Ongoing education and collaboration with the family Consistent collaboration with the interprofessional team **In patient referral for:** In-hospital schooling Social worker for family support **At discharge:** Community outreach support	**Presents to the emergency department with parents in family vehicle.** **Nurses' role on admission:** Secure IV access points Haemodynamically stabilise child Pain relief Wound care Arrange transfer to tertiary paediatric centre Provide initial support and education to the family Consistent collaboration with the general practitioner **At discharge from tertiary centre:** Support with ongoing wound care School nurse support **Referrals for:** Community nurse or GP practice support

a   Present and explain your preferred context of care to a small group.

b   Describe what opportunities you would have in each context of care to expand your scope of practice.

	Tertiary Burns Unit	Rural Emergency Department
Preferred context of care and why		
Scope of practice opportunities in each area		

4.5 National Health Priority Areas

The National Health Priority Areas (NHPAs) of health care need have been identified as the most prevalent and as having the most impact on the population and the national health care budget; that is, they carry the greatest burden of disease. Currently there are nine **National Health Priority Areas** (see Figure 4.4).

National Health Priority Areas
Priority health care areas identified as significant for the Australian population.

While all of these areas of health care are identified as a priority, some health care environments show more prevalence than others. For example, injury is noted to be more prevalent in males, people over 65 years, Aboriginal and Torres Strait Islander peoples and those who live in remote areas of Australia. Asthma is more common in Aboriginal and Torres Strait Islander peoples, the older adult age group and people living in socioeconomically disadvantaged areas. It is therefore in your best interest to research the health care sector where you seek employment so that you are clearly aware of, and prepared for, the context of care in which you will work and the levels and priority area in which you will be providing care.

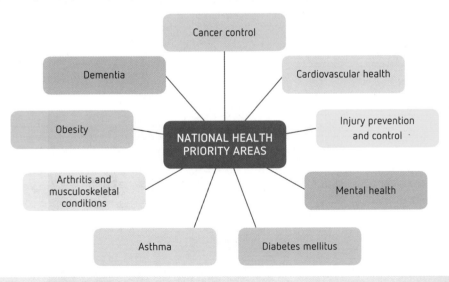

▶ Figure 4.4 National Health Priority Areas

PRACTICAL APPLICATION: PREVALENCE AND HEALTH CARE SECTORS

In small groups, examine the three NHPAs below and, focusing on the available government data, show the prevalence of the priority area in each sector.

Discuss and explain why there may be differences in the prevalence for each health care sector.

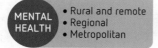
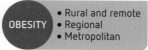
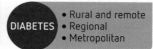

HOW DID YOU GO?

Were you able to identify if there were any differences in the health care data for those people living in the different areas? This type of exercise helps you to value that being an RN is not a 'one size fits all' occupation. Nursing is a profession that can take you in any direction that you wish to go. You do, however, need to be conscious of opportunities and how to embrace them.

FOCUS POINTS AND MOVING FORWARD

Regardless of where you work, nursing will place physical, emotional and cognitive demands on you. It is therefore important that you find your own space, where you feel that you can work effectively and positively as an RN. There are significant career choices and opportunities when working as an RN, and the Australian health care environment will provide you with many opportunities of different types and levels of practice. Do not be limited to only those contexts of care that you experienced on clinical placement. Use those experiences as a springboard to other aspects of health care. Think about where your patient may have been transferred from or where they may be referred to for ongoing care. Be always mindful of the changing contexts of care, for example, hospital in the home, and how changes in health care policies and guidelines may lead you to another health care experience.

DISCUSSION POINTS

1. Role-modelling is a very powerful method to promote health and wellbeing in others. Discuss how you would role-model healthy behaviours to your nursing peers to encourage them to maintain a healthy lifestyle.

_____

_____

_____

_____

2. Discuss the scope of practice differences that could be expected for an RN in Australia. Consider those of experienced RNs working to their full scope in practice in a regional hospital's emergency department to that of an RN working in a regional centre's child health clinic.

_____

_____

_____

_____

3. The National Health Priority Areas are described in the terms of 'burden of disease.' Define this term and discuss how the nine National Health Priority Areas are a burden of disease to the Australian population and economy.

_____

_____

_____

_____

REFERENCES

Bishop, L., Ransom, A., & Laverty, M. (2017). _Health care access, mental health, and preventative health: health priority survey findings for people in the bush._ Royal Flying Doctor Service of Australia. https://www.cwaa.org.au/images/PDF/RN032-Healths-Needs-Survey-Result.pdf

Edelman, C., & Kudzma, E. (Eds.). (2018). _Health promotion throughout the life span_ (9th ed.). Elsevier.

Kearney-Nunnery, R. (2020). _Advancing your career – concepts of professional nursing._ FA Davis Company.

Naidoo, J., & Wills, J. (2016). *Foundations of health promotion*. Elsevier.

Tveiten, S. (2021). Empowerment and health promotion in hospitals. In G. Haugan & M. Eriksson (Eds.), *Health promotion in health care – Vital theories and research* (1st ed.). Springer International Publishing.

USEFUL WEBSITES

National Health Priority Areas (NHPA), https://www.countrysaphn.com.au/community/national-health-priority-areas

Population Density (June 2018). Australian Bureau of Statistics, https://www.abs.gov.au/ausstats/abs@.nsf/Previousproducts/3218.0Main%20Features602017-18?opendocument&tabname=Summary&prodno=3218.0&issue=2017-18&num=&view=#:~:text=Australia's%20population%20density%20was%203.3,square%20kilometre%20(sq%20km)

The Australian Health System, Australian Government Department of Health (last updated 2019), https://www.health.gov.au/about-us/the-australian-health-system

National Strategic Framework for Chronic Conditions (last updated 2020), https://www.health.gov.au/resources/publications/national-strategic-framework-for-chronic-conditions

Australian College of Nursing, Career Hub, https://careers.acn.edu.au

Australian College of Nursing, Nursing Now, https://www.acn.edu.au/nursingnow#:~:text=About%20Nursing%20Now,of%20nursing%20around%20the%20world

CHAPTER

5 PREPARING FOR THE CHANGING HEALTH CARE ENVIRONMENT

Learning objectives

Working through this chapter will enable you to:

1. adapt to changing health care equipment and systems
2. recognise the need to maintain competencies with technological advances in the rapidly changing health care environment
3. identify the nurse's role in public health and primary health care
4. engage with the role of leadership in nursing to enable a culturally safe and fair health care environment
5. incorporate self-awareness, social awareness and situational awareness as a catalyst to expand your scope of practice in the changing health care environment.

Introduction

Nursing sits within an environment that is forever changing. With the development of new understandings and philosophies of health care, the changes in people's health care needs and the advancement of resources and technology, every decade places nursing in a new position of practice. Also, the increasing use of health promotion strategies has afforded a health care environment where infection rates, fatal injuries and cancers are in the decline. As a result, people can live longer and healthier lives. A significant negative change, however, is the increase in non-communicable diseases caused by behaviours such as unhealthy diets, reduced exercise and stress-related lifestyles. This has created a population of people living with chronic conditions, which demands a new approach to nursing care.

As a graduate registered nurse (GRN) entering the health care environment, it is important to remember that changing health care needs will shape your learning, and it does not stop once you receive your university degree parchment. Your area of practice will challenge you to become an expert in that area and the ongoing changes and improvements to practice will demand that you keep up with the new clinical guidelines from an evidence-based approach to care.

5.1 The changing Australian health care system

The drive to address our population's health care needs through research and development is facilitated with funding from governmental and private organisational groups. Large numbers of research projects are always in place, with the aim to not only reduce health care costs, but to improve the quality and length of life of the world's population (Australian Institute of Health and Welfare [AIHW], 2021). There are also significant efforts made to create and adapt equipment that is more intuitive, limits or stops errors in patient care and reduces the need for human resources. These are regularly introduced into the health care sector. Much of this equipment you will have seen and used in the health care environment during your clinical placement experiences, where you would have been closely supervised. As a graduate the expectation is that you will be able to independently utilise health care equipment, such as patient monitors, volumetric pumps, hospital beds and computer-based systems so that you can provide the highest level of care for your patients (Ferguson, 2021).

Working within your scope of practice is paramount here, because if you are unfamiliar with a device and cause harm to the person in your care or to the device itself, you will need to take responsibility for the harm caused as well as be accountable for the outcome. It is perfectly reasonable, therefore, to ask for assistance and guidance when you are faced with an unfamiliar piece of equipment. This does not excuse you from not proactively recognising new equipment in your clinical environment and seeking to understand its purpose and function. Descriptions of most pieces of medical equipment can be found on the internet with published videos and written materials and your clinical facility will have manuals and equipment documents.

While this may sound worrying, lifelong learning and ensuring that you stay abreast with changes in the health care system on all levels is a fundamental role of the RN. Most clinical facilities will alert you to any changes in their area. It is then up to you to utilise any in-service training opportunities so that you are able work within those changes. Be alert to the introduction of new equipment into your clinical area and be aware of any workshops or information sessions that will assist you in expanding your scope of practice in this area.

PRACTICAL APPLICATION: HEALTH EQUIPMENT AND PROFESSIONAL STANDARDS

You may think that as an RN you do not need to understand how the health equipment you use works effectively, or be able to recognise when it is malfunctioning or is unsafe for use. You may also think it is not your responsibility to critically assess whether it is even necessary to use the equipment to meet the patients' health care needs. This could not be further from the truth. All seven standards for practice need to be met when using health-related equipment.

a   In small groups, discuss each of the seven standards for practice listed in the table in relation to using health equipment in direct patient care. For each standard for practice, provide an example of the type of equipment (e.g. patient lifting equipment, such as hoists or slings) and a situation where you have experienced or witnessed this equipment.

Registered nurse standards for practice	Example of equipment	Situation experienced or witnessed
1. Thinks critically and analyses nursing practice		
2. Engages in therapeutic and professional relationships		
3. Maintains the capability for practice		
4. Comprehensively conducts assessments		
5. Develops a plan for nursing practice		
6. Provides safe, appropriate and responsive quality nursing practice		
7. Evaluates outcomes to inform nursing practice		

HOW DID YOU GO?

In your discussions were you able to identify how you need to apply each of the standards of practice when using health equipment with patients in your care? Did it make sense that you need to assess the situation and your patient's needs before starting or continuing to use the equipment? Was using a critical approach to care and ensuring that you developed a trusting relationship central to the discussions about safe practice?

5.2 Being part of the data revolution

The implementation of the digital health records system has provided an opportunity where enormous quantities of **data** can be gathered and analysed. This system helps government and organisations see the trends and patterns of health and illness that relate to current practices. On a national scale, it is easy to see waiting times in emergency departments, numbers of missed infections causing delayed discharge, readmission due to early discharge and the statistics of medication errors. It also makes clear what practices are working best and therefore need to be championed, maintained or augmented. The opportunities that this data offers for further research is endless and in turn will drive further change and practices into the future. The Connecting Australia to a healthier future webpage provides more information about how the digital health systems currently in place in Australia are utilised (see the list of useful websites at the end of the chapter). There is a dedicated portal for health care providers to give you more specific information to help you prepare for practice.

data
Information in the form of facts.

There is a variety of digital software and hardware used in the health care space in Australia. The Australian Institute of Health and Welfare (AIHW, 2022) lists technologies such as mobile devices to send text reminders for appointments and for health-related applications (apps), electronic discharge summaries and the My Health Record database. Other types of **technology** may be **telehealth** consultations for patients

technology
Devices used to support health care practices.

telehealth
Health care provided using technological devices.

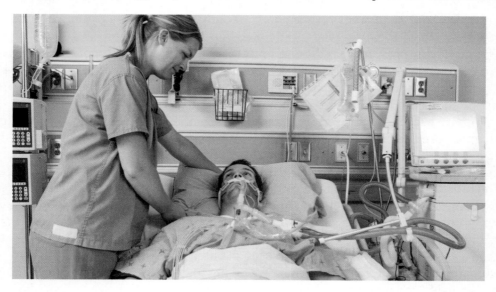

Source: Shutterstock.com / Tyler Olson

in outlying areas, smart watches, electronic prescribing devices, wearable devices and robotic nurse assistants. The technological advancements are rapid and focused on reducing costs and providing best patient care. As a lifelong learner working in contemporary health care, you will be expected to work effectively with these devices as part of your changing practice responsibilities.

You will have also noted when on placement that health care facilities often use their own software platforms to record patient data and to manage their health care needs. As a GRN, it is important to not let these platforms become an obstacle in your transition to practice. Gather as much information about them as you can as early as possible, even when you are first offered the role. Ask about the platform and if they have a 'sandbox' that you can practice with. It's important that you master these programs quickly as you will be working with them every shift, and to have a computer program delay you unnecessarily is frustrating for everyone.

5.3 Public health changes to nursing practice

health promotion
Empowering people to take control of their health and wellbeing

The domain of public health is one where the population is considered from a position of **health promotion** and disease prevention. Public health services collect data and look for trends and changing patterns that may be damaging to public health or changing the focus of current health care practices. The responsibilities of the public health arm in Australia are very broad and span from reviewing sanitation services to predicting population growth and health care service needs (Keleher, 2020). Reviewing AIHW webpages, such as Health promotion and health protection, and health promotion textbooks (e.g. Edelman & Kudzma, 2018) will demonstrate the need for health care to be from 'a whole of population' approach. This means all people (across the lifespan) are supported to empower them to healthier living.

Primary health care nurses are often the first point of contact with a community and must use the opportunity to create an environment of empowerment and self-efficacy (see Table 5.1). The aim is to promote health and wellbeing by encouraging people to adopt healthy lifestyles while also incorporating health-derived medical screening tests and self-management health care strategies into their life routine. For example, the nurse's role in enabling self-management was prominent when supporting people through the COVID-19 pandemic. Nurses needed to ensure that people understood isolation and quarantine expectations and that they would know when to seek further assistance. This augmented the already increasing role of autonomy of the RN, with more nurses working in community settings facilitating healthy living and quality of life goals across the whole of the Australian population.

As a GRN working in a primary health care role, you need to be alert to the changing trends and behaviours of the environment you are working in and use

▸**Table 5.1** Primary health nurse roles

Primary health nurse roles	
Community health nursing	Rural health nursing
Community mental health nursing	Occupational health nursing
Maternal, child and family nursing	Nursing in general practice
School nursing	Home based nursing
Your health nursing	Correctional nursing
Sexual health nursing	Nurse practitioners
Alcohol, tobacco and other drugs nursing	

Source: adapted from Guzys et al., 2017.

this knowledge to adapt and inform the health promotion needs of the community. It is therefore important that you communicate openly with the people in your care and be very aware of the materials and resources that inform and influence the behaviour of those around you. This may be information from social media, websites, magazines, television and newspaper reports. These are the materials that will influence behaviours in your community, and you do need to be aware of these influences in your practice.

5.4 Global health and the Australian health care system

Prior to the COVID-19 pandemic, international travel was a common phenomenon. With millions of people moving across the globe at any one time, the transference of pathogens between countries was nonchalantly accepted as 'you always pick something up on a plane'. As an island, and prior to cost effective travel options, Australia was generally protected from large tourism movement. In recent decades, though, increasing tourism in Australia, Australia's immigration policy and the seeking of skilled workers from other countries, has generated a change in the demographics and numbers of people living in Australia seeking health care services (AIHW, 2018). It is important to remember that these newcomers will have experienced other types of health care systems, may have witnessed or been directly exposed to war and violent conflict, perhaps had a lifetime of inadequate nutrition and health care and may have been separated from family and friends. Also, dietary changes can pose difficulties for new arrivals to Australia who may find that foods common to their table are not easily found or are expensive. Remember that the physical and mental health wounds that accompany immigrants and refugees to Australia may not be obvious, so it is essential that you bring **cultural safety** to your care when working with all people so that everyone feels supported (Power & Usher, 2021).

global health
An approach to health care that is worldwide.

cultural safety
Creating an environment where everyone feels safe, respected and valued.

diversity
The differences between people that make us unique individuals.

As a GRN, remember that **diversity** comes in all forms, and you will be constantly working with a diverse group of people whether in a work or a home environment. We all have different upbringings, levels of education, beliefs and values. Accepting and embracing differences should be celebrated and is a valuable opportunity to learn from the experiences of others.

REFLECTION: THE CHANGING IMAGE OF THE NURSE

The global COVID-19 pandemic has demonstrated how a single virus can bring catastrophic changes on an international scale. The need for nursing care has never been greater and the thousands of images of nurses from every country in the world in full personal protective equipment (PPE) highlights the importance of this large workforce of health care professionals.

a   In your groups, discuss how the public image of nurses has changed globally.

b   Describe how nurses' public health roles expanded during the COVID-19 pandemic and how nurses were instrumental in enabling public health safety standards to be introduced and maintained.

c   Write a reflective statement on how this pandemic/public health experience impacted on your career choice to be a nurse.

HOW DID YOU GO?

The COVID-19 pandemic was the first time in history that a virus could be tracked with such detail and accuracy. Previously, herd immunity was the only recourse, but this time, waiting in lockdown-type environments with regular testing to determine where lockdowns were to occur until a vaccine was created, was a new alternative. The nurse's role was, and is, one of solidarity and support for the community as a whole. Nurses deliver care with calm, compassion and concern. Did you resonate with this image of the professional RN?

The nurse as leader in a changing world

It is during times such as the COVID-19 pandemic where the nurse can lead the community through health care challenges. Clinical nurses are in a unique position of working directly with the people in their care. This enables the nurse to keep abreast of patient needs and changing trends in the patient's world as it unfolds. This unique perspective is well recognised by the collaborative health care team who aim to work seamlessly with an RN to ensure that patients receive holistic care that is cognisant of global health and community health needs.

leadership
An approach to nursing practice that influences others to bring about change.

These **leadership** roles of change agent, collaborator and advocate place you, as the GRN, in the ideal position to realise and initiate care within the changing health environment (Ferguson et al., 2020). This does not mean that you will be changing laws or organisational policy in your first year of practice, but it does mean that you must be alert to changing practices and be aware of issues of practice or anomalies that may be impacting on your ability to provide best practice and act upon them.

If you witness issues of health inequality and health inequity it is an expectation of culturally safe practice that nurses advocate to ensure that all people feel respected and valued, and they have the opportunity to access health care that meets their needs (Ward & Tham, 2020). Health equality is when everyone is treated the same way, regardless of their situation. Much like asking a fish to climb a tree, you can't expect a person who needs a wheelchair for mobility to be able to climb stairs. This becomes an health equity issue – one of justice and fairness. You must, therefore, be alert to situations where the person in your care may be disadvantaged due to limited resources and limited consideration of their needs.

5.5 Scope of practice changes in a changing environment

Working within your scope of practice is fraught with complexity in the everchanging world of health care in Australia. As a GRN, just when you think you have found your feet and are able to meet the demands of your workplace, a new situation pops up for you to reconsider. For example, you may be promoted to another position or be tasked to care for someone who has a health problem that is outside of your scope of practice. If this occurs, the principle of working within your scope of practice, regardless of the environment of care, applies and you need to be very confident in what areas of practice you will need support and direction in.

It is your ability to assess your own needs through **self-awareness**, to identify team interactions through social awareness, and to determine the 'big picture' through situational awareness that will enable you to move forward to a position of confident knowledge-seeking in any health care environment. Value your changing care environments, by documenting and recording all skills and learning opportunities so that you can demonstrate your continuity of professional development. This information will be needed for you to demonstrate to the regulatory body your motivations and ability to learn from your environment of practice. Refer to the Nursing and Midwifery Board's (NMBA's) continuing professional development (CPD) fact sheet to see what is expected of you to maintain your registration and how you can best do this, by drawing from your practice experiences as a catalyst for learning (see Figure 5.1).

> **self-awareness**
> Awareness of your own needs, growth and ability to change.

Date	17/5/23	23/5/23	30/5/23
Source or provider details	NMBA	Advanced life support in practice (XYZ Provider)	Obstetric emergency training (XYZ Provider)
Identified learning needs	RN Standards for practice Practices in accordance with legislation affecting nursing practice and health care.	NA	NA
Action plan	Clarify responsibility for aspects of care with other members of the health team. Unsure of my delegation responsibilities in the workplace. Plan: Access and review decision-making framework.	NA	NA
Type of activity	Self-directed learning. Review of NMBA decision-making framework	Workshop	Workshop
Description of topic(s) covered during activity and outcome	Reviewed my scope of practice and the scope of practice for my profession. Understood the principles I need to apply when making decisions about my nursing practice and when and how I decide to delegate activities to other RNs and ENs.	Advanced Life Support re-accreditation	Obstetric emergency re-accreditation
Reflection on activity and specification to practice	This activity has enabled me to achieve my learning need as per my learning plan. As a team leader working in intensive care, I will be able to apply the Nursing decision-making framework when I allocate staff to patient care and delegate tasks as they arise during a shift.	This activity provided me with new theory and a practical competence assessment in relation to advanced life support. I will be able to apply this to patients in respiratory/cardiac arrest and when part of the medical emergency team.	This activity provided me with new theory and a practical competence assessment in obstetric emergencies.
No./Title/ Description of evidence provided	Refer to item 6	Refer to item 7 Certificate of attendance	Refer to item 8
CPD hours	2 hrs	3 hrs	3 hrs

Source: The Nursing and Midwifery Board of Australia (NMBA)

▶ Figure 5.1 Sample template for documenting CPD

PRACTICAL APPLICATION: PROMOTING CHANGE AS A GRN

a   Reflect on your clinical experiences. Identify one thing that you believe could be changed for the better. It may be a very small change to practice that you think will impact the care of and comfort for your patients, or it may be a generic change that would need escalating to enable a policy review.

_____

_____

b   In small groups, discuss your point for change. Select one that you all agree on.

_____

_____

c   Referring to the steps below, write a plan for how you, as a GRN, could draw attention to the need for change and facilitate this change.

_____

_____

_____

_____

Steps to raise awareness of the need for change
Understanding and clarifying the needed change. (What and why?)
People who would need to be involved to enable the change. (Who?)
Planning the process to raise awareness of the need for change. (When and how?)
Implementing the strategy to raise awareness for change.
Evaluating the effectiveness of the plan to promote change.

HOW DID YOU GO?

As a nurse leader there is an expectation that you will be consistently looking for situations where change is needed to promote best practice. You do, however, need to consider and be mindful of all aspects of the problem or issue before going forward. Involve all stakeholders and discover if this problem has been addressed previously and, if so, why it has continued. You are looking for barriers so that you can be creative in your problem solving.

FOCUS POINTS AND MOVING FORWARD

The rapid changes in health care and the global trends of disease processes provides a fundamental repositioning of the nurse's scope of practice, employment and practice options. The need for changes in practice are also influenced by digital health records in Australia, which provide a national image of health care needs and services. It is the understanding of the health care environment from a broader scope that enables you, as an RN, to understand the trends and changes that are occurring in your own health care environment. This will assist you to prepare for changing needs in the population as a whole, which will mean changes in treatment plans and new equipment developed to improve care options.

DISCUSSION POINTS

1. Consider health care equipment that you have used in the clinical environment. Discuss how you ensured that the patient, rather than the health care equipment, was central to the care provided.

_____

_____

_____

_____

2. Advocating for a culturally safe and equitable environment is a central leadership role of an RN. Discuss this point.

_____

_____

_____

_____

3. Discuss how situational awareness is an important skill to identify changes in the health care environment.

_____

_____

_____

_____

REFERENCES

Australian Institute of Health and Welfare. (2018). *Culturally and linguistically diverse populations. Australia's health 2018*. Australia's health series no. 16. AUS 221. Canberra: AIHW. https://www.aihw.gov.au/getmedia/f3ba8e92-afb3-46d6-b64c-ebfc9c1f945d/aihw-aus-221-chapter-5-3.pdf

Australian Institute of Health and Welfare (2021). *Health system overview*. https://www.aihw.gov.au/reports/australias-health/health-system-overview

Australian Institute of Health and Welfare (2022). *Digital health*. https://www.aihw.gov.au/reports/australias-health/digital-health

Guzys, D., Brown, R., Halcomb, E., & Whitehead, D. (Eds.). (2017). *An introduction to community and primary health care* (2nd ed.). Cambridge University Press.

Ferguson, C. (2021). Technology and professional empowerment in nursing. In J. Daly & D. Jackson (Eds.), *Contexts of nursing* (6th ed., ch 13, pp. 223–239). Elsevier.

Ferguson, C., Newton, P., & Edwards, J. (2020). Clinical leadership. In E. Chang and J. Daly (Eds.), *Transitions in nursing. Preparing for professional practice* (5th ed., pp. 227–236). Elsevier.

Keleher, H. (2020). Public health in Australia. In E. Willis, L. Reynolds & T. Rudge (Eds.), *Understanding the Australian health care system* (4th ed., pp. 71–84). Elsevier.

Edelman, C., & Kudzma, E. (Eds.), (2018). *Health promotion throughout the life span* (9th ed.). Elsevier.

Power, T., & Usher, K. (2021). Cultural safety in nursing and midwifery. In J. Daly & D. Jackson (Eds.), *Contexts of nursing* (6th ed., pp. 335–348). Elsevier

Ward, B., & Tham, R. (2020). Rural health systems: spotlight on equity and access. In E. Willis, L. Reynolds & T. Rudge (Eds.), *Understanding the Australian health care system* (4th ed., pp. 136–154). Elsevier.

USEFUL WEBSITES

Australian Safety and Quality Framework for Health Care, https://www.safetyandquality.gov.au/sites/default/files/migrated/ASQFHC-Guide-Healthcare-team.pdf

Australian Institute of Health and Welfare (AIHW), Health system overview (updated 2021), https://www.aihw.gov.au/reports/australias-health/health-system-overview

AIHW, Health promotion and health protection, https://www.aihw.gov.au/reports/australias-health/health-promotion

Nursing and Midwifery Board of Australia, Registered nurse standards for practice, https://www.nursingmidwiferyboard.gov.au/Codes-Guidelines-Statements/Professional-standards/registered-nurse-standards-for-practice.aspx

Connecting Australia to a healthier future, Australian Digital Health Agency, https://www.digitalhealth.gov.au

Fact sheet: Continuing professional development. Nursing and Midwifery Board of Australia, https://www.nursingmidwiferyboard.gov.au/codes-guidelines-statements/faq/cpd-faq-for-nurses-and-midwives.aspx

PROACTIVELY PREPARING FOR YOUR TRANSITION TO PRACTICE AS A GRN

Learning objectives

Working through this chapter will enable you to:

1. discover how the health care team is a valuable resource to support the graduate registered nurse during their transition to practice
2. prioritise and capitalise on having a strong understanding of the procedures of practice and the documentation standards that are expected of the registered nurse in the clinical facility
3. communicate effectively with the health care team using paper and digital documentation
4. demonstrate the significance of knowing where to locate resources and clinical equipment to ensure care is timely and efficient.

Introduction

The Australian graduate registered nurse (GRN) is baccalaureate prepared to work as a beginner in any health care environment where registered nurses (RNs) are employed. Due to the diversity of nursing positions across Australia, your clinical placement experiences would have introduced you to a very small sample of health care facilities, and you may find yourself employed in an unfamiliar clinical environment (Australian Institution of Health and Welfare [AIHW], 2018, Section 2.1). You will probably be unfamiliar with the people in the health care team, the unique procedures of practice required, the documentation expectations and the layout of the health care facility. Do not be worried as many before you have experienced the same situation, and with some general principles of preparation you will be able to transition into your new area of practice quite quickly and without duress.

6.1 The people: colleagues and consumers

colleagues
Other health care professionals who nurses work with.

It is the **colleagues** you work with who will be your initial supports, and it is therefore essential that you take the time and make the effort to find out who they are. Some health care areas have a large number of nursing staff (e.g. >150 nurses) so it will take time to get to know many of them by name and face. So, start by knowing who the nursing staff are on your shift. Find out their role and allocation and note it down on your planner. This means you can approach nursing team members by name and start to develop a **network** of support for yourself. Also, identifying each person's areas of expertise or strengths will give you a resource base to draw upon during your shift. This will save you time and provide you with relevant and accurate information to enable you to work confidently to your scope of practice.

networks
A grouping of like-minded people who support each other.

Hospitals

Understanding how medical teams function in your acute clinical environment can be confusing initially, as public and private health care hospitals have different admitting rights for medical personnel. For example, a primary level hospital in a rural area will have general practitioners (GPs) who admit patients to the hospital, whereas large metropolitan public hospitals will have hospital-employed specialist doctors who are the only ones with admitting rights. Private hospitals in regional centres may allow both GPs and specialist doctors to admit patients. In general, tertiary centres have large teams of medical doctors, and it will be the resident medical officer (RMO) who is usually your first point of contact. In a private hospital it is the private doctor that the patient is 'admitted under' who is your contact for medical advice. Where possible, check the medical roster so that when you do call you know the RMO/GP/doctor by name and face if they come to the ward area. Making this effort will enable you to build **rapport** and open communication channels with other medical personnel as quickly as possible.

rapport
A connection between people that is underpinned by empathy and understanding.

You will work with many other allied health care professionals, administrative personnel and IT support staff employed by the hospital, as well as people external to the facility, such as clergy, community nurses and community allied health care professionals. You will also be communicating regularly with food service staff, cleaning staff and at times tradespersons doing plumbing, electrical and carpentry work if needed. Your ability to know who the people are in your clinical environment, what they do and why they are there, will be essential for you to understand how they relate to or can be supportive of you when providing care.

Community and clinics

You will find that community-based and primary health care environments will have different health care teams, which will be dependent upon the consumers' needs and the health care sector. For example, a school nurse may work closely with an educational psychologist, an occupational therapist and the local GP. If in a community service that supports people with drug and alcohol problems, nurses will be working with counsellors, social workers, medical specialists, psychologists, dieticians and the nurses specialising in those areas. Getting to know the names of people in the team and their roles and responsibilities gives you a head start to working collaboratively to ensure health care goals are set and met.

Seeking advice and assistance

Seeking assistance from the interprofessional collaborative health care team is one area that new graduate nurses often express as challenging. Working within your scope of practice, knowing the recommended escalation procedures and being very confident of your patient's clinical situation, is essential when you are seeking support from another health care professional. Using a framework, such as **ISBAR** (introduction, situation, background, assessment, recommendation; see Figure 6.1; SA Health, 2016), which is a highly flexible mnemonic tool that can be used in any form of clinical handover, will allow you to present your information logically and in a format that will allow the health care professional to understand your request or concerns. Plan this out before you make the phone call or approach the health care professional. Be sure to have all the relevant information and assessment data, as it wastes time if you need to run off to get information.

ISBAR
A mnemonic tool that can be used in any form of clinical handover, which stands for introduction, situation, background, assessment, response/requirement.

I

INTRODUCTION
Introduce yourself, your position in the clinical area, and the patient in your care and give their name, age, gender, diagnosis and any information that you think will 'set the scene'.

S

SITUATION
Describe briefly why you have called; for example, the patient has fallen, has had a surgical intervention and is complaining of intense pain, was admitted to the ward three hours ago due to …

B

BACKGROUND
Describe relevant past medical history and anything that you think is relevant to the current situation; for example, Mr X has a medical history of cardiovascular disease diagnosed 10 years ago and type 2 diabetes diagnosed three years ago …

A

ASSESSMENT
The assessment should be as recent as possible and include vital signs as well as a focused assessment specifically related to the situation. For example, if the patient fell, then you would assess for mobility issues, pain, skin integument damage, as well as considering the cause for the fall, such as medications, inappropriate foot wear, etc.

R

RESPONSE/REQUIREMENT
It is very important that you state what you need. For example, do you need a doctor to come and undertake a medical assessment; do you need a medication order over the phone; do you need some advice or direction; do you need to arrange for the patient to be admitted to the ward from the emergency department or to return from the operating theatre? Don't expect the other person to guess what you need. You have to state this clearly.

▸ Figure 6.1 ISBAR

Working with the collaborative team

Do not forget that the collaborative team is a highly valuable resource and support system for you as a GRN. Taking the time in the early days to introduce yourself to the allied health care professionals (AHCPs), will save you a lot of time and angst over knowing who to contact in certain situations. As you introduce yourself, seek information about the AHCP's role and responsibilities in your area of practice. Ask how often they attend the ward, how they can be contacted, if they are involved in the team meetings, and if you can call on them if you have a question. Knowing this information will, again, save you a lot of time and confusion over knowing your best point of contact. Of course, you will have support from nursing personnel that you should always draw on if needed, but including the other members of the health care team expands the support that is available to you.

PRACTICAL APPLICATION: THE INTERPROFESSIONAL TEAM

List five different health care professionals who you may work with in an interprofessional collaborative team. Describe their roles and responsibilities and how their knowledge and expertise would assist you as a beginner in your role as an RN.

_____

_____

_____

_____

_____

HOW DID YOU GO?

Who you chose as your health care professionals is probably reflective of your clinical experiences. Did you already know their roles and responsibilities, or did you need to search for this information? Were you able to identify discipline-specific areas of health care that each health care professional could assist you with?

6.2 The processes: professional and organisational

When you were on clinical placement, you may have found that the Nursing and Midwifery Board of Australia's (NMBA's) professional standards and codes of conduct were interpreted and applied slightly differently in each clinical area and were dependent on the needs of the people seeking care. The breadth of standards is intentional as it provides the nurse with the flexibility needed to ensure that care is individualised and person-centred. This breadth of application can be disconcerting, however, for the GRN who is just starting to develop a sense of assurance of practice. What is important is that as a beginner you work within the standards and codes and use them as guidelines for best practice. For example, think of the NMBA guidelines as the white lines on a road. You can drive anywhere within the guidelines but not outside of them, unless you are making a definite change. It is the same with the NMBA standards for practice and codes of conduct. They provide you with a breadth of reasoning and decision making so that you can be flexible and creative in the care you provide.

It is therefore very important to be cognisant of the standards for practice and the policies and codes that guide you. These resources provide you with guidelines that will assist you when determining your scope of practice and how to work professionally within the health care environment. For example, advice in relation to social media use, the Australian Charter of Healthcare Rights from the Australian Commission on Safety and Quality in Health Care, and working within the International Council of Nurses' Code of Ethics for Nurses provides you, as an RN, with valuable resources and guidelines that will not only keep the public safe but also keep you safe in your practice (see list of useful websites at the end of the chapter).

Differences between facilities

clinical guidelines
Guidelines that guide the nurse in the care of a patient.

Remain mindful that different facilities may have adapted or written their own **clinical guidelines** for the provision of care, have different patient admission or health assessment procedures and have different expectations of you as a GRN. For example, in some clinical areas you will be allocated a number of weeks of supernumerary time with another RN, whereas in other clinical areas it maybe one or two days. Others will expect you to take on a full patient load from the outset and expect you to seek advice and support when needed, and others will provide you with a smaller load, for example, 50 per cent, and increase this incrementally dependent upon your level of confidence.

Differences between health care professionals

It is also important to remember that all health care professionals work within their own discipline's standards for practice and codes of conduct. While some of the codes may be similar in many areas, and collaborative patient-centred care is common, it is not appropriate to assume that all health care professionals are guided by exactly the same regulations. It is also important to realise that each discipline's scope of practice will vary, so take the time to review and aim to understand the role and responsibilities of the health care professionals you are working with and their scope of practice before making a request. To make unreasonable demands of others in the health care team does not enable a collaborative approach to practice as it is judgemental and makes assumptions of their practice expectations (Slusser et al., 2019).

Human resources considerations

When working as an RN, there will be other processes to be very mindful of. This includes understanding the submission of a timesheet and understanding the pay roll system for your clinical facility. Don't assume that you will be paid the same rate as a beginning RN in all facilities as some are known to pay different hourly rates and they may also have a different promotional scale process. Be mindful that if you work in a nursing position where you do not accrue shift rate bonuses, your fortnightly pay will be significantly different to those who do. Also, working in rural and remote areas may be accompanied with financial incentives and assistance with accommodation and transport. Review documents such as the Pay Guide – Nurses Award from the Fair Work Ombudsman (to see how the pay system works when working public holidays, on the weekend and outside of business hours) and the nursing and midwifery salary guide from Queensland Health to understand superannuation processes and salary packaging (see list of useful websites at the end of the chapter). Knowing when you will be paid, how you will be paid and what mechanisms are in place to ask questions about aspects, such as long service leave, will set you in a good space for your financial security.

Understanding the rostering system

Understanding the rostering system will provide you with more opportunity to have choices in your life and to achieve a work–life balance. Finding out if you can request specific shifts, knowing how far in advance the roster is developed and if you can 'bank' days off, will be an opportunity to shape your own preferences into the roster (see, for example, Australian Nursing and Midwifery Federation Northern Territory, n.d.). Other important points to understand are the Australian taxation system and what deductions you can make in relation to uniforms, textbooks and equipment needed to perform your job (see Figure 6.2). Having a sound understanding of these rules and laws will provide you with the knowledge as to where options and opportunities can add to your quality of working life.

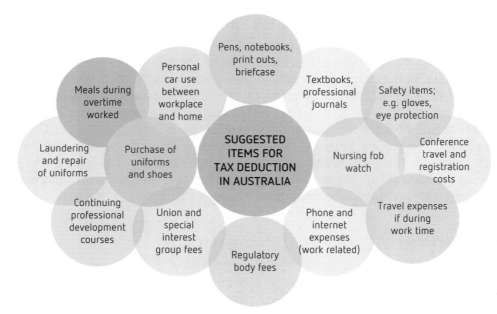

Meals during overtime worked

Personal car use between workplace and home

Pens, notebooks, print outs, briefcase

Textbooks, professional journals

Safety items; e.g. gloves, eye protection

Laundering and repair of uniforms

Purchase of uniforms and shoes

SUGGESTED ITEMS FOR TAX DEDUCTION IN AUSTRALIA

Nursing fob watch

Conference travel and registration costs

Continuing professional development courses

Union and special interest group fees

Regulatory body fees

Phone and internet expenses (work related)

Travel expenses if during work time

▶ **Figure 6.2** Suggested items for tax deduction in Australia

PRACTICAL APPLICATION: INFORMAL MENTORING

A good way to understand the processes of your clinical facility is to raise points for discussion (e.g. intranet, rostering, policy documents) with the other members of the health care team.

a   List what information about the procedures or processes you would like to know more about in your clinical area or nursing in general (e.g. professional development).

_____

_____

_____

b   Write a short script as to how you would raise this point with a colleague.

_____

_____

_____

_____

c   In groups of three, role-play the interaction and gain feedback as to the effectiveness of the interaction.

_____

_____

_____

_____

HOW DID YOU GO?

Were you able to identify some key processes that you will need to be very aware of when transitioning into your role as a GRN? Was it difficult to find the correct language to use when approaching someone for advice and their experiences? Do you think that the role-play gave you a sense of confidence when pursuing these areas of nursing practice?

6.3 The paperwork: documentation and documents

As an RN, the responsibility to document accurately and in a timely manner falls squarely on your shoulders. Often, written documentation is the only way to communicate with other health care professionals. If you fail to document or wait too long to update, then other health care professionals may miss vital information that would otherwise inform their clinical decisions. Remember that the care of your patient is not just nursing care, it is from the position of all members of the collaborative health care team. If the nurse does not provide accurate and timely feedback or information, the patient's care could be compromised.

Documentation: being accountable

It is timely to remind you, that you are accountable for what you document (Australian Commission on Safety and Quality in Health Care, 2022). You will no longer have your progress notes countersigned by another RN. Therefore, if another health care professional asks you about a point that you have made in a patient's notes, you will need to respond to their questions and back up your statements with a comprehensive explanation. Remember that 'if it is not documented it is not done' and it is not acceptable to add in material or delete/erase what has already been written. The rule of putting a line through an error and signing it reinforces that a patient's progress notes are a legal document and must be treated accordingly. The message is: do it right the first time. Write draft copies (remember to shred these) until you are satisfied that the information is succinct but informative, accurate and has enough description that any health care professional will clearly understand your report. Also, work on developing your own **routine** and style of documentation. This enhances your competency and accuracy when documenting and leads to meeting the expectations of the nursing profession in your own way.

routine
Behaviours and tasks that are so well practiced they become second nature.

Electronic documentation platforms

With the introduction of My Health Record, which is the national electronic health record, into the Australian health care system, as well as some sectors continuing to use paper-based systems, you will need to be flexible and actively learn the different formats. When you were on placement, you would have noted that there were many different types of documents for different situations. It can be very time consuming trying to find the correct document in the health care environment and it may even delay a patient's discharge or treatment plans. Therefore, develop your knowledge of the documentation system of your workplace as early as possible. See if the hospital has an intranet site where the documents are filed, so that you can familiarise yourself with them off shift or during your orientation. Ask if you can take images of the paper-based forms. Locate and understand how to complete forms that you may not need to use regularly, such as mother admission with baby documentation, a medication error, a death on the ward, incomplete documentation, progress notes or any other unique forms. Also find out the process for when the electronic health record system fails – what happens then? Make lists of common documents you will use so you can work more independently early in your graduate year.

Remember that, generally, all documentation is looking for the same outcome, it is just that some documents are more detailed than others and are from a different perspective. A comprehensive assessment and a clear plan for your patients' care needs and processes should be the basis for all documentation.

6.4 The plan: layout of the immediate health care environment

Knowing where to find things in the ward should not be underestimated. As already noted, knowing the people you work with, the processes you will work from and the paperwork that you will need to complete are essential for a smooth transition to practice. It is also essential that you can efficiently and effectively locate resources, people and equipment in your ward area as well as the organisation itself. It is therefore important in your first few days of practice to diligently develop an overall plan as to where to find things. This can range from linen to medication to documents to wheelchairs. Being able to quickly find things not only will increase your sense of belonging and understanding of the resources in your environment, but it will also enable you to use your time more effectively and not delay a patient's care. In an emergency situation, it can mean providing care quickly rather than waiting for five minutes while the necessary equipment is found.

Being consistently mindful of your environment places you in a position of power and control over your planning, where you are always alert to changes to the environment and where to find resources. Test yourself. See how quickly and accurately you can find things. Go to your shift 20 minutes early and look in cupboards, in trolleys and on the hospital system. Create an image in your mind of the pattern of where you find the closest hand basin, IV pole or fire extinguisher.

You also need to know where to find facilities outside of your ward area as often you may need to go to these departments or direct patients to them. When you have received a notice of your employment, go to the hospital or facility and take a walk around. See if you can find the X-ray and ultrasound departments, the pharmacy, the rehabilitation area, the education centre and library, operating theatres and ICU, and the cafeteria. Knowing the location of other departments and facilities provides you with location awareness and adds to your sense of autonomy by being able to go to departments effectively and efficiently from the beginning of your graduate year. You can also confidently direct others who will see you as interested and motivated in your place of work.

PRACTICAL APPLICATION: KNOWING YOUR CLINICAL ENVIRONMENT

a   Draw a floor plan of a current or previous clinical placement area that was in a large hospital/clinical facility.
b   Make a list of the resources or physical spaces that you would need on a single shift to provide patient care.
c   Show these on your floor plan.
d   Now draw a plan of the hospital/clinical facility itself showing departments and areas where you either needed to visit or to direct patients to.
e   Find other students who have drawn the same hospital/clinical facility and share your drawings to check for accuracy.

HOW DID YOU GO?

Drawing the floor plan of the clinical area should have been straightforward enough, but when you were drawing the hospital, were you able to identify emergency parking, the security offices and food services areas? Directing people to the nearest café or park or shopping centre that is outside of the hospital grounds is valuable, especially for those families who have been relocated from rural and regional centres.

FOCUS POINTS AND MOVING FORWARD

This chapter looked into the different environments in which you will be working. Be aware that there are many different places of practice for RNs. Read widely to see what may be available to you so that you can make an informed career choice. Do not consider nursing to be stagnant or that your practice will never be changing and dynamic. Grow your career by being forever mindful of available opportunities and engage with the people and the practices in the environment in which you work to enable your expertise to grow and develop.

DISCUSSION POINTS

1. The interprofessional collaborative team provides a positive environment of rapid learning for the GRN. Discuss this point.

    _____

    _____

    _____

    _____

2. Discuss how, as a GRN, you can utilise resources, such as the clinical facility's intranet footprint, to familiarise yourself with the priorities and goals of the facility.

    _____

    _____

    _____

    _____

3. Discuss and develop a plan of action that enables you, as a newcomer to a clinical facility, to develop a sense of belonging and confidence in your practice.

    _____

    _____

    _____

    _____

REFERENCES

Australian Commission on Safety and Quality in Health Care. (2022). *Documentation of information*. https://www.safetyandquality.gov.au/standards/nsqhs-standards/communicating-safety-standard/documentation-information

Australian Institution of Health and Welfare. *Australia's health 2018*. https://www.aihw.gov.au/getmedia/f2ae1191-bbf2-47b6-a9d4-1b2ca65553a1/ah16-2-1-how-does-australias-health-system-work.pdf.aspx

Australian Nursing and Midwifery Federation Northern Territory. (n.d.). *Rules of rostering*. https://www.anmfnt.org.au/resources/rostering

SA Health. (2016). *ISBAR A standard mnemonic to improve clinical communication*. Safety and Quality Unit. https://www.sahealth.sa.gov.au/wps/wcm/connect/8a8b26804896068a9cb8fc7675638bd8/15111.3-+Clinical+Handover+Fact+Sheet+%28V1%29WebS.pdf?MOD=AJPERES&CACHEID=ROOTWORKSPACE-8a8b26804896068a9cb8fc7675638bd8-nwKWYoN

Slusser, M., Garcia, L., Reed, C., & McGinnis, P. (2019). *Foundations of interprofessional collaborative practice in health care*. Elsevier.

USEFUL WEBSITES

Australian Charter of Healthcare Rights, ACSQHC, https://www.safetyandquality.gov.au/consumers/working-your-healthcare-provider/australian-charter-healthcare-rights

International Council of Nurses, The ICN Code of Ethics for Nurses, https://www.icn.ch/system/files/2021-10/ICN_Code-of-Ethics_EN_Web_0.pdf

My Health Record, Queensland Government, https://www.health.qld.gov.au/system-governance/records-privacy/my-health-record

Nurses Award, Fair Work Ombudsman, https://www.fairwork.gov.au/employment-conditions/awards/awards-summary/ma000034-summary

Nursing and Midwifery Board of Australia – Social media: How to meet your obligations under the National Law, https://www.ahpra.gov.au/Resources/Social-media-guidance.aspx

Wage rates – Nursing Stream, Queensland Health, http://www.health.qld.gov.au/hrpolicies/salary/nursing

PART 3

FINDING YOUR PROFESSIONAL SPACE

Learning outcomes

1. Be confident of your career goals and professional preferences and how to work towards those.
2. Understand how to apply professional practice guidelines and policies to become the expert registered nurse that you want to be.
3. Understand how best to examine the health care environment to enhance your professional development as a beginning registered nurse.

Preamble

The attrition rates of graduate registered nurses (GRNs) continue to add to the ongoing nursing shortages worldwide. Accurate figures are difficult to obtain as many nurses move to part-time work or take a break from employment for study and maternity/paternity leave, while others maintain their registration meeting minimal requirements when they are unsure of their ongoing career plans. Nursing offers a breadth of employment opportunities that people in other careers are not able to even imagine. Your choice is therefore one of opportunity, availability, forward planning and being practice ready to achieve your career goals. Remembering that you may need to gain experience from several areas before you can reach your final goal is important. Therefore, as a GRN you should think carefully about your preferences for employment, your need for postgraduate study and then plan strategically to meet your short- and long-term goals

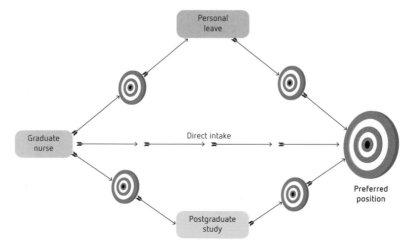

7

FINDING THE BEST RN GRADUATE POSITION FOR YOU

Learning objectives

Working through this chapter will enable you to:

1. understand that 'organisational fit' is a vital component for you as a graduate registered nurse to consider when selecting your employment
2. develop your professional portfolio
3. actively and strategically look for employment opportunities that meet your needs and preferences
4. identify and apply transferable experiences when finding your professional space
5. engage with opportunities for professional development and career progression.

Introduction

Finding your preferred nursing role as early as possible in your career is a valuable steppingstone to achieving job satisfaction and fulfillment. However, not finding your 'dream job' as a graduate isn't an impediment to your long-term goals as a registered nurse (RN) as having an expanded scope of practice provides a broader scope of understanding and employability. You can capitalise on your varied experiences and develop a career goal that meets your needs and your preferences.

7.1 Organisational fit: what fits best for you?

As nurses we readily take a safe person-centred approach to care, but to work as a safe and effective RN, you need to be very conscious of your own professional and personal needs and advocate for them within your role. Working tired, stressed or distracted poses safety risks to yourself as well as your ability to provide care, and has been shown to impact on nurses' sense of achievement and fulfilment. Therefore, finding an organisation that is willing to understand and meet your needs by supporting you in your work is paramount to achieving job satisfaction and to maintaining a commitment to your goals.

Some graduates may state that they 'just want a job'. And while this is understandable after three long years of very demanding university study and clinical placement expectations, it is not the attitude that you should carry with you for the long term. If you see nursing as 'just a job' you will soon find the cognitive and physical demands of the work to be overly taxing and you may look for something more 'you'. It is important then that you identify early on what it is that is 'you'.

7.2 Growing your professional portfolio

portfolio
A file or compendium that stores experiences for the nurse in their growth and development as a professional.

Developing and maintaining a comprehensive professional **portfolio** that houses your files of assessment pieces, journaling, feedback from clinical support staff and reflections of your clinical experiences will assist you in moving towards the RN that you wish to become. At university, your assessment results are housed in your academic history, and while it does show your overall score, it does not show how you learnt, what were the major influencing factors in your learning progression or your musings about where you are going to go from here. As a student, the portfolio provides you with a resource where you can showcase your learning trajectories, how you are moving towards areas of speciality or particular interest and, importantly, your ability to become a lifelong learner. A capability which is an expectation in the standards for practice (Nursing and Midwifery Board of Australia [NMBA], 2016) and highly sought after in the health care industry.

Do not think of your portfolio as only necessary for your student years. In fact, your registration can only be maintained with the support of examples of

continuing professional development
An expectation of learning (rated in points) that establishes the nurse's currency of practice.

recency of practice
Nursing practice (rated in hours) that demonstrates that the nurse is up to date in their clinical practice capabilities.

continuing professional development and **recency of practice**. This evidence of being up to date needs to be recorded and provided if the NMBA seeks to audit your ability to meet ongoing registration standards. Keeping a portfolio of your professional development record and practice hours as a GRN and all the way through your career as an RN is very important proof of your ability to meet mandatory registration standards for practice.

Your portfolio does not need to be overly complex or cumbersome. In fact, the easier it is to pinpoint your experiences as a resource to inform career progression, the better it is. It can be in the form of a spreadsheet, a blog or vlog site, or even an audio repository. There are also many apps that you can download to your smartphone to record your experiences and learning opportunities every week. What is important is that you engage with your portfolio at least every two to four weeks. What you put in the portfolio will be driven by your aspirations, your experiences and where you see your professional career taking you (Smith & Cusack, 2021). For example, if your aim is to be a diabetes

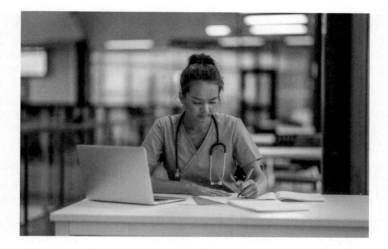

Source: iStock.com/FatCamera

Consistent forward planning enables you to put your qualifications and experiences to use

nurse educator, then your experiences in diabetes or experiences in education should be your focal point. While you do not ignore other clinical experiences, concentrate on those areas of practice that will take you to where you want to be. Presenting your experiences so that they are in a logical and understandable format is essential. For example, you may like to develop a framework that helps you log your experiences that demonstrate how your professional practice and knowledge is progressing. Revisit and tweak your plan so that it remains realistic and achievable and use it as a benchmark as to how you are tracking towards your career goal.

PRACTICAL APPLICATION: GIVE YOUR PROFESSIONAL PORTFOLIO SIGNIFICANCE WITH A 'STATEMENT OF INTENT'

Create a cover sheet for your professional portfolio and write a 'statement of intent' on the cover. This statement should outline your purpose for becoming an RN. To get started, think about why you studied nursing in the first place. There must have been something that stood out for you. What kept you studying and going to your placements?

Try to narrow down to the essence of why you want to work in nursing. Rather than, 'I want to make a difference in someone's life', think about the actual difference you were thinking of. How would you make that difference, what role models you have found along the way to give you absolute direction and which patient group or demographic were you aiming to help?

It is these types of questions that will enable you to centre your thinking about your career and professional progression, as it will give meaning and purpose to your study and guide you toward your professional career goals.

HOW DID YOU GO?

Were you able to fine-tune your intention to study nursing? Did you find that you had limited analysis behind your intention in your first years of study, but can now add more depth and reasoning?

Your statement of intent may not be something that you discuss with your peers, but if you have a family member or friend who you value as a mentor, explore your intentions with them. Lateral thinking may assist you to uncover hidden reasoning behind your choice. This in turn may provide you with a solid foundation of professional goals in which to base your career progression.

7.3 Finding the place where you can grow and be the RN you want to be

Now that you have thought broadly about your career preferences, you need to find a professional space where you can express these aims, and professionals who will actively support you to move towards your career goals. As a student you will have had the opportunity to observe RNs working in many different roles and situations. Reflecting on those role models is paramount to your beginning professional development and to facilitating your changing identity to that of an RN. Taking on aspects that you saw as excellent practice and sophisticated professional behaviours are foundational to your career development and will pave the way towards your aspirations and preferences in practice.

Choosing the organisation and context of care in which you want to practice (i.e. community, acute, paediatric, rural) is your starting point. Link this with a particular geographical place or health care sector and you can start to piece together your preferences for practice. Or, think about the areas of practice that you least prefer (i.e. adult but not acute care; regional but not community; aged care but not independent living). This will help you narrow your choices in your search for your GRN position and beyond.

PRACTICAL APPLICATION: PROFESSIONAL PREFERENCES AS AN RN

a   Complete the table below by listing your first three preferences of where you would like to work as an RN: geographical space (e.g. city/rural/country); the health care sector (e.g. primary/secondary/tertiary) and the type of health care (e.g. surgical/paediatric/community/chronic). Don't think too hard about it. Just write down what comes first into your mind.

b   In small groups, discuss your choices and explain why you chose those areas of nursing practice. If you can explain these to someone else, then your choice will start to take shape in your mind, or you may realise that there is more thinking to be done. Once you have clarified and validated your professional preferences, add them to your professional portfolio for future reference and guidance.

Geographical space	Health care sector	Type of health care

HOW DID YOU GO?

This activity is valuable as it gives you the opportunity to choose something and examine it carefully. You may find that it is not your preference after all, but it will help you to navigate opportunities and see your way forward in your nursing career.

Aligning your values and goals with an organisation of choice

Considering your preferences and what you value in nursing and then aligning these with an organisation's values and beliefs is another method in which to seek out a workplace that may be your best 'fit'. All health care facilities offer a mission or philosophy statement, a core values statement or identify their organisation's goals and aims on their website. Be sure to review these carefully in your search for organisational fit. Also, think about what you would like to achieve in your short- and long-term plans and see if your goals align with the organisation's goals and achievements. Particularly look at how they support their staff for these achievements to occur.

By seeking out and carefully reading through the information that the organisation provides, you will have a better understanding of their values, intentions and strategies when it comes to providing best patient care, and how they would support you in your career development. This will help you seek out an organisation where you will feel valued and welcomed, and where your career goals will be validated and nurtured. It will also add to your confidence when you present these aligned values and goals at your job interview.

REFLECTION: COMPARING YOUR VALUES AND GOALS TO THAT OF A HEALTH CARE FACILITY'S PHILOSOPHY AND/OR MISSION STATEMENT

a   List your own career values and goals using the table below as a guide.
b   As a group, visit the website of one of the health care facilities that group members would like to review as a possible place of employment. List the organisation's stated values and goals and compare these to your preferences.

c   Discuss these in your group from the position of being employed in that workplace. Decide on the potential organisational 'fit' in relation to your values and the feasibility of you working there in order to meet your goals.

GRN professional preferences	Organisation
Your values	Organisational values
What you want to achieve (goals)	The organisational achievements (goals)

HOW DID YOU GO?

Did you locate the health care facility's values and goals and could you identify with those? If you did not, then think about why you were unable to 'gel' with the organisation's aims. Look further at other health care facilities and see if they are more in line with your professional thinking.

7.4 Finding employment as a GRN outside of the usual health care venues

The role of the nurse is ever developing and changing and is influenced by many factors. These factors can be driven by new disease processes that change models of care, more sophisticated investigation and treatment management plans, societal expectations and population growth. It can also be government driven with health policies, National Health Priority Areas, budget allocations and financial projections all impacting on the changing role of the nurse. These factors greatly influence how nursing positions will grow and be funded.

Look outside of your clinical placement experiences and those mainstream health care services that are familiar to you (see Figure 7.1). As a nurse you may find valued and satisfying nursing work in areas of practice such as primary health care

RN EMPLOYMENT OPPORTUNITIES	CARING FOR VULNERABLE POPULATIONS	WORKING AS AN RN IN OTHER COUNTRIES
Hospital facilities	Mental health	Developed countries
Community facilities	Aged care	Developing countries
Primary health care facilities	Disability care needs	Countries in extreme poverty
Correctional facilities	Homelessness care needs	Countries supporting refugees
Defence force facilities	Domestic violence care needs	Countries recovering from war
	Aboriginal and Torres Strait Islander peoples	

▶ **Figure 7.1** Examples of the breadth of nursing employment opportunities

in correctional centres and the defence forces. You could also work in community support settings with our most vulnerable populations needing nursing care, such as organisations that support people with disabilities, mental health concerns, homelessness and domestic violence. So do not limit your options to only those you saw as a student of nursing. Consider the opportunities that nursing offers to travel and/or to bring about a change of lifestyle.

Working abroad

As an Australian RN, your registration will also allow you to work in many different countries, and while most graduates seek to work their first year of practice in the Australian heath care system, some have used it as an opportunity to begin their practice elsewhere. Countries such as New Zealand, Papua New Guinea, South Africa, the United Kingdom, Ireland, Canada and some Middle Eastern and European countries recognise the NMBA's nursing registration for employment. Other countries such as the United States, however, require a licensure pass in their National Council Licensure Examination (NCLEX) before commencing practice. While you will need to seek out specific details from each country's own regulatory body, the Australian website Health Times provides you with some resources to start thinking about expanding your nursing career options in another country (see the list of useful website at the end of the chapter).

Remember also that there are many opportunities to work as an RN in developing countries. This is an excellent way for you to gain a perspective on how health care can be and is practiced in different health care environments. Experiences such as these cement your ability to apply theory to practice as you are often working in busy environments where health care services can be limited. Here you will become a flexible problem solver and work in many different contexts of care with a rapidly expanding scope of practice. If you are thinking about this approach to gaining experience in your nursing career, there are many organisational websites that will provide information about these services. Two examples of organisations that encourage nurses to join them in humanitarian relief programs are UNICEF and the Australian and International Red Cross. If you are interested, read all the information carefully so that you are aware of the expectations, as well as the housing and support you would receive.

Being openminded and holistic in your search for employment

Your ability to network and connect with others who are or have been in a similar situation to yourself is an excellent method to gain further insights into how other people are working towards achieving their career goals. Be mindful, though, that while this information is very valuable and gives you a benchmark or a target in which to work towards, you should always approach this information with a realistic open mind. Just because one person wants to work in a particular area of practice in a particular country to gain **promotion** in a certain area, does not mean that you must do the same. The competitive nature of the human mind can cloud your own thinking and may sway your view away from what is important to you. Return to your reflective journals and your portfolio of study and clinical experiences. What did you enjoy the most and why? Think about where you would happily go to work every day and feel as though it was your space; a space in which to grow your knowledge and skills. This has to be your **vision** as to where you can become the best possible RN that you can be.

promotion
Moving to a different level of expertise within a discipline of practice.

vision
Imagining a concept or environment of change.

Using transferable knowledge and skills to gain employment

The transfer of skills gained from previous employment experiences outside of nursing are well accepted and valued by the recruitment team when reviewing applicants for a beginning RN position. When considering **transferable** skills and knowledge, the focus is often on communication, teamwork and leadership. And while these are all valued essential skills in the health care system, think beyond the superficiality of the skill to the depth of the strengths that you can bring to the health care environment. For example, being the captain of a sporting team holds different leadership skills to being the manager of a supermarket team. Consider the responsibilities that you held in your previous role(s) and draw from those skills to support you as you transition into nursing practice, and as you think about your career progression. Which of those transferable skills can be developed further in nursing so that you become an **expert** in an area of practice? How will these skills propel you forward to your career goal? What skills and knowledge can you present in your job application and interview to demonstrate the quality of your strengths?

transferable
The ability to move skills and knowledge gained in one area to another clinical area or discipline.

expert
A person who has high levels of knowledge and skills in a particular clinical area or discipline.

REFLECTION: WORKING WITH YOUR STRENGTHS IN YOUR SEARCH FOR A GRADUATE POSITION

a   Think about one of your skills that you feel you have developed well. Write this skill in the space below. It may be something you are skilled at because you have practiced it many times in a non-nursing area, or you have a particular interest in it and have read about it widely, or you have had the opportunity to practice it often during your clinical placement (e.g. open mindset, taking neurological observations, attending to hair hygiene).

b   Focus closely on each of the strengths that are associated with this skill and list them in the table below. Complete the other columns so that you can articulate how your existing and transferable strengths will assist you in your transition to practice as an RN.

c   Add this table to your professional portfolio. Then write a short paragraph responding to this job interview question: 'Please identify one of your strengths and explain how this strength will support you in your transition to practice as a GRN'.

Skill: _____

_____

What are the strengths associated with this skill?	How will each of these strengths empower my transition to practice as a GRN?	How could these strengths be developed further in my nursing career?	How will these strengths propel me to my career goal?

HOW DID YOU GO?

Your strengths may come in many shapes and forms, some of which you may even be unaware of. It is, therefore, always useful to ask others for their observations of your skills, professional attitudes and behaviours, and ability to meet the professional standards of practice. You do not have to agree with the feedback you receive, but it is always important to take from it that which is useful to you as a way of improving your practice. If you gain feedback that is not helpful or constructive, then it may not be worth examining in any depth.

7.5 Forward planning and your career development

As an early career RN, positioning yourself to be in the right place with the right qualifications and experience at the right time to achieve promotion takes planning, skill and often luck. Knowing when a role will become available can be quite easy to determine if you know that some staff are planning retirement, taking leave or moving to another position. Being **proactive** and ready is the best way to ensure that when a role becomes available you have the necessary prerequisites to apply for it (see Figure 7.2). You can achieve this by working towards recognising and developing transferable skills and experiences, and by seeking out and completing relevant courses, workshops and postgraduate programs that will pave your way forward. Join special interest groups, and attend conferences, workshops and seminars that will demonstrate your commitment to your career goal and will, in turn, develop your professional network.

proactive
Anticipating and acting on a need or situation before it occurs.

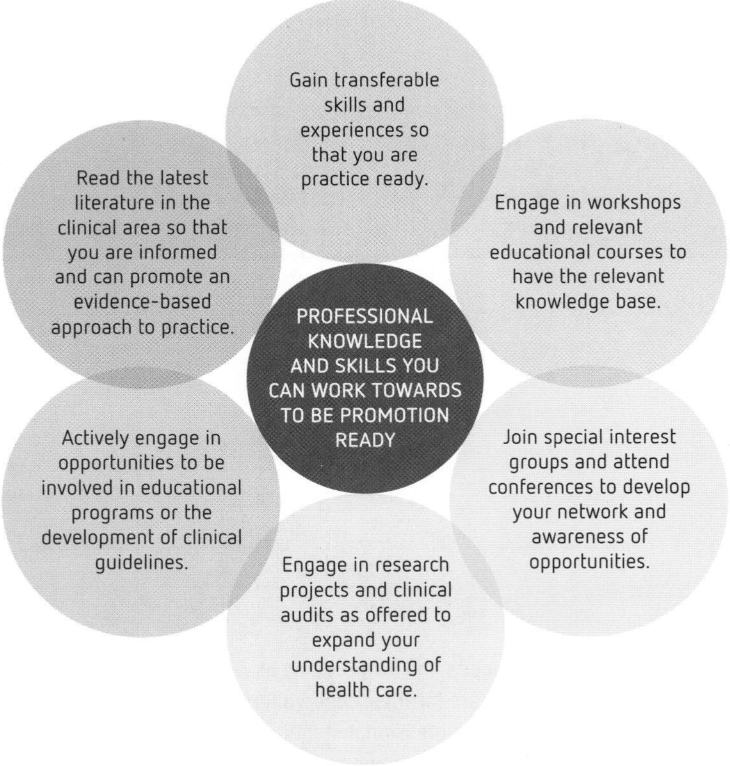

Gain transferable skills and experiences so that you are practice ready.

Read the latest literature in the clinical area so that you are informed and can promote an evidence-based approach to practice.

Engage in workshops and relevant educational courses to have the relevant knowledge base.

PROFESSIONAL KNOWLEDGE AND SKILLS YOU CAN WORK TOWARDS TO BE PROMOTION READY

Actively engage in opportunities to be involved in educational programs or the development of clinical guidelines.

Join special interest groups and attend conferences to develop your network and awareness of opportunities.

Engage in research projects and clinical audits as offered to expand your understanding of health care.

▶ Figure 7.2 Planning for promotion as an early career RN

Also engage in research projects, clinical audits or other opportunities, such as assisting with educational programs or clinical guidelines as they become available. All these activities indicate your desire to be a professional RN who is prepared to gain the necessary skills, knowledge and experience to achieve their career goal.

Taking the long road may be the best road

Seek to understand where there is an abundance of GRN positions in a particular area. These areas will provide you with less competition and increase your likelihood of achieving a position. Graduates are often keen to work in areas such as emergency departments and intensive care units, and while it is important to have a goal, there are limited places for GRNs in these areas and you may find that you will need to take a diverted route to achieve this goal. If this is the case, be sure that your career plan is flexible and able to cope with deviations and time delays. Be prepared to travel or move to other parts of the country or the world to gain the experience you may need. Look to regional centres where employment vacancies are often noted to be more prevalent than in metropolitan areas, and consider what postgraduate study you may need to complete to help you towards your goal.

Even if you have a clear vision of your career goal, be prepared for the path to not be as straight or predictable as you had envisaged. The phrase 'being in the right place at the right time' is certainly one that has influenced nurses' careers in the past. For nurses who are in the right place at the right time, they may quickly move towards their goal, but for others the opposite can occur if the availability of positions or a redirection of funds changes the employment landscape. While this may be frustrating and an irritation for you, it is important to realise that there are always other options. Think broadly – is it your path that needs to divert to bring you back on track, or does your goal itself need to shift slightly? Do you need to take a completely different path altogether? Remember, it is your journey, so make it happen the way you want it to (see Figure 7.3).

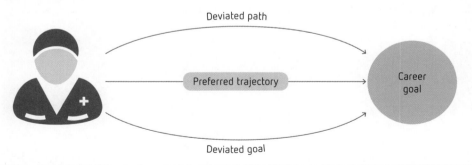

▶ Figure 7.3 The path to your career goal

FOCUS POINTS AND MOVING FORWARD

While most organisations look closely to see if you will 'fit' their organisation, you should also be asking if that organisation is the best 'fit' for you. Ask yourself, will they provide me with the best opportunities for learning, job security and career development? Will I be able to develop my existing strengths and be supported in areas that are outside of my scope of practice? Will it be my vision and my goal that I am working towards here? Considering these points will provide you with a point of self-advocacy where you are focusing on your preferences and your needs. This will lead you to a career that is satisfying and rewarding as you move towards being an expert RN.

DISCUSSION POINTS

1. Discuss the role of the nurse and why it is appropriate that employment in nursing is so diverse.

_____

_____

_____

2. All GRNs are supported in their area of clinical practice. Discuss the areas of nursing practice where you think you will need the most support.

_____

_____

_____

3. Consider the concept of promotion. Discuss how being acknowledged through promotion could improve the retention rates of nurses.

_____

_____

_____

REFERENCES

Nursing and Midwifery Board of Australia. (2016). *Registered nurse standards for practice*. https://www.nursingmidwiferyboard.gov.au/codes-guidelines-statements/professional-standards/registered-nurse-standards-for-practice.aspx

Smith, M., & Cusack, L. (2021). Developing a professional portfolio. In H. Harrison, M. Birks, & J. Mills (Eds.), *Transition to nursing practice: From student to professional* (Ch 3). Oxford University Press.

USEFUL WEBSITES

Australian Primary Health Care Association, https://www.apna.asn.au

Defence Jobs, https://www.ncsbn.org

Health Times, https://healthtimes.com.au/working-abroad

Unicef Australia, https://www.unicef.org.au

Australian Red Cross, https://www.redcross.org.au/about/how-we-help/international-aid

Nursing and Midwifery Board of Australia, Recency of practice, https://www.nursingmidwiferyboard.gov.au/registration-standards/recency-of-practice.aspx

Nursing and Midwifery Board of Australia, Continuing professional development, https://www.nursingmidwiferyboard.gov.au/registration-standards/continuing-professional-development.aspx

Nursing and Midwifery Board of Australia, Audit, https://www.nursingmidwiferyboard.gov.au/registration-and-endorsement/audit.aspx

National Health Priority Areas, https://www.health.gov.au/sites/default/files/australia-s-long-term-national-health-plan_0.pdf

CHAPTER 8

MORPHING INTO THE RN YOU WANT TO BE

Learning objectives

Working through this chapter will enable you to:

1. analyse your goal and set a realistic starting point when working towards your career and professional development
2. appraise your own career goals and strategies
3. initiate mentorships with people who can guide you through your early career
4. proactively advocate for a learning pace that enables retention and best practice as a beginning practitioner
5. debate the importance of self-care and healthy living so that you can practice as a registered nurse effectively and safely.

Introduction

As a beginning health practitioner, you are looking forward to becoming a confident and autonomous registered nurse (RN) who works from a position of evidence, and who can independently engage with the health care team to ensure the person in your care is safe and feels well cared for. And while this is an excellent goal, it will take some time for you to get to this point and is best supported by a realistic approach, which is flexible and open to deviations along the path. Do not rely on others to 'tap you on the shoulder' or to give you career progression advice. It rarely happens. So, it is up to you to seek out information, mentors and people who will support and guide you on your way to becoming the RN that you want to be.

8.1 Identifying a realistic starting point

Thinking ahead to the professional RN and expert that you aim to be is a fundamental step in your career development; however, having a realistic view of where you are at the moment is equally as important. Knowing where the professional 'you' currently sits on your goal trajectory gives you an excellent starting point. You can form this realistic view by honestly thinking about your scope of practice for your clinical area, your level of knowledge and capabilities, your understanding of what is expected of you as an RN and how this will change as your career progresses. Starting off with over-inflated and unrealistic beliefs about your knowledge and abilities means that you do not have, and will not seek out, the foundational material that you need to progress. Conversely, having an undervalued or an underdeveloped understanding of your knowledge and experience as a beginning RN means that you could be simply 'marking time' and not progressing as you should if you had a more accurate understanding of your professional self.

Working as an RN: ideas and aspirations

Nursing is a profession that has many dimensions and if you were asked to define nursing, you would probably focus on the tasks you do, the people you care for and the knowledge that underpins these things. Therefore, the nursing roles you aspire to are limited only by your understanding of the roles and responsibilities that RNs can hold in different contexts of care and areas of practice. For example, you are probably aware of the primary care roles and responsibilities of a school nurse, but there are also primary health care nurses who are linked with organised camping programs, film sets, amusement parks, and large sporting events, such as the Commonwealth and Olympic Games. There are nurses who do not work as clinicians but as advisors for governmental bodies, who help write policies and advise teams who are investigating and advocating for change in the health care system. RNs can work for private insurance companies examining insurance claims, or work in telehealth providing support and care to those people who do not have local health care services. There are nurse navigator clinicians who help people with chronic complex conditions find suitable services in the ever-expanding health care system, and also occupational health and safety nurses working in factories and industries. The breadth of opportunities for RNs is immense; however, as a student you may have only worked with nurses in specific clinical facilities and observed nurses working in academia, so your aspirations may be limited. Read widely and explore the many positions available to you as both a graduate RN (GRN) and an experienced RN (see also Table 8.1). Knowing what is out there provides you with a dynamic platform of opportunity on which to base your professional decisions and choices.

▶ **Table 8.1**   Nursing opportunities that you may not have considered

Health care sector	Suggested nursing roles within each sector
Primary health care	Practice nurse – GP or specialist School nurse Community health nurse Correctional services nurse Aged care nurse Rehabilitation care nurse Palliative care nurse
Advisory roles	Clinical advisor – aged care Legal health nursing advisor Continence / diabetes nurse advisor Insurance nurse advisor Pharmaceutical company nurse advisor Health government nurse advisor Nurse navigator / case manager

Health care sector	Suggested nursing roles within each sector
Occupational health nursing roles	Factories Businesses; e.g. airports Mining sites State police service Remote area medical centres Nurse immuniser Youth detention centres

8.2 Foreseeing nursing positions

One fundamental approach to looking for employment as an RN is to see where the government's health budgets are being directed. Examining documents such as the National Health Priority Areas and action plans such as the National Men's and National Women's Health Strategies 2020–2030 provide valuable information as to where current and future funding will be allocated to support the Australian community. Other documents, such as Securing Australia's Nurse Workforce from the Australian College of Nursing, are valuable resources to see firsthand the direction that health care will be taking for the Australian RN. If you add those to other resources that identify where nurses are working and in what numbers, for example, the Health Workforce Data from the AIHW, you can gain insight into where positions are available and where opportunities are likely in the future. Gaining this solid understanding will allow you to grow and progress towards your career ambitions. See the list of useful websites at the end of the chapter.

PRACTICAL APPLICATION: CAREER PROGRESSION PLAN

a   List your top career goal; for example, to gain the role of Clinical Nurse Consultant in a community health clinic within five years of full-time work as an RN. Describe how your current scope of practice will support your progression to your goal. Then, using the table below as a guide, add to each column how your scope of practice needs to be expanded and developed to achieve the goal. In the bottom row write how your progression plan is realistic, feasible and achievable.

b   Once this is completed, discuss with your class group how you determined that your plan was realistic. Be sure to recognise that while something may be realistic to one person it may not be to another, and there always needs to be flexibility and open mindedness in your planning.

Career goal: _____

_____

Grad. Year 1	Year 2	Year 3
Scope of practice	Scope of practice	Scope of practice
Realistic	Realistic	Realistic
Feasible	Feasible	Feasible
Achievable	Achievable	Achievable

HOW DID YOU GO?

You may have found that the breadth of career goals that your classmates expressed was quite wide. It will depend very much on each person's personal goals as well as their professional goals. A focus on travel, beginning a family or undertaking postgraduate study will place very different focal points on a nurse's career direction. Stay true to yourself and focus on what you want to achieve.

8.3 Developing your expertise through mentorship

Your graduate year is an excellent time in which to seek out a mentor who can guide and support you in your early transition stages to becoming an RN. There are many definitions for the term **mentor**, but generally as a graduate commencing your nursing career, it is someone who can guide you towards your career goal (Fontaine et al., 2021). There are no rules as to who a mentor can be. It may be an expert clinician working with you on the floor, it may be a formally designated support person, or it could be a friend or relative who you find easy to talk to and can help you think about things from a number of perspectives.

mentor
A person who guides or directs another.

Mentoring is about you and your needs, so when you seek out a mentor, think about what you wish to gain from the relationship so that you can progress your career. Do you need someone who is an expert nurse who can help you think clinically about your progress and your experiences, or do you need someone who

PRACTICAL APPLICATION: FINDING THE BEST MENTOR FOR YOU

a   In your class groups, discuss the characteristics of a professional and personal mentor. Then discuss, as a mentee, what professional attitudes and behaviours you would need to bring to a mentoring meeting to enable an effective outcome.

b   Draw mind maps, like the ones shown, to help you complete this task.

c   In pairs, role-play a mentor–mentee interaction with the mentee bringing predetermined goals and concerns to the meeting.

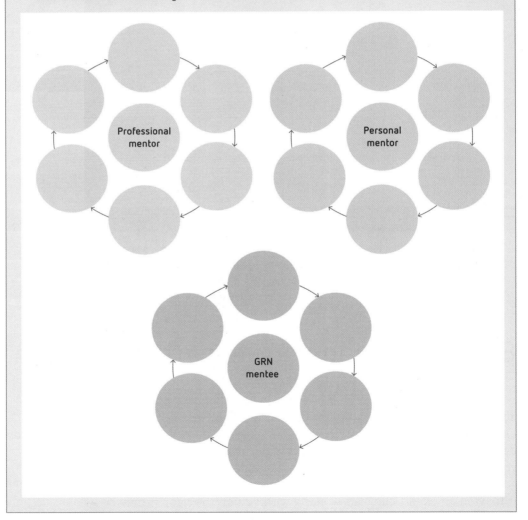

> **HOW DID YOU GO?**
>
> A strong, honest and trustworthy mentor is invaluable, so it is worth the effort to seek out someone who understands you as a person and as a professional. Do not be disheartened if you do not connect well with your first mentor. Keep looking and find that person or those people who inspire and support you.

can assist you to think about the bigger picture, such as how to achieve a work–life balance. Remember that a mentor can be someone who you have not formally asked or who has been allocated as a mentor. They may be someone who you observe in the workplace and use their professional behaviour as a guide, acting as a silent mentor (Woolnough & Fielden, 2017), or someone who you catch up with occasionally to have a chat with, acting as an informal mentor. Either way, this is about you and your career progression, so you must bring clear goals and objectives to the mentor–mentee relationship. Do not wait for the other person to suggest a meeting or set an agenda, it is your career, and you need to make this work. You also need to document these meetings and the outcomes of each, as well as where you want to go with the next one. These should be clearly described in your professional portfolio and recorded as a reflective paragraph after each meeting.

8.4 Learning as a GRN

Learning is of course central to your career development and becoming the RN that you aspire to be. In the first few months as a GRN, you will find that learning in the clinical area will be almost constant as new and different experiences come your way. What is important is that you 'pace' your learning and you do not allow this large input of information to overwhelm you. Your **short-term memory** can only hold a certain amount of data before you become **cognitively saturated**, and you will not be able to retain or recall things easily or at all (Donovan et al., 2021). This is when mistakes can happen, or you may forget to do something.

learning
An event where information is applied to previous knowledge.

short-term memory
Information that has been recently stored for quick retrieval.

cognitive saturation
A situation when the short-term memory is unable to store any more material.

You need to take control of the learning and demands that are placed on you. There are a number of strategies that you can use to do this (see Table 8.2). One important point is to not rely on your memory (even for the smallest thing), take brief notes and add to them and reread throughout your shift. Another strategy is to stage your learning by asking to care for the same patients over a number of shifts so that you can consolidate your previous knowledge and perfect your clinical skills. Take some time when you are off shift to reflect on the patients' medical conditions and treatment needs so that you become more confident with each care opportunity.

▶ **Table 8.2**   Enhancing learning through workload monitoring

Strategies to reduce cognitive overload	Workload strategies to enhance learning
Ensure that your shift planner is checked and updated regularly (hourly at a minimum).	Care for the same patients so that you can build on your experiences from previous shifts.
Make a 'to do' list even for the smallest tasks.	Advise your team leader if the workload is too great as early as possible.
Note points to be followed up.	Arrange support for tasks outside of your scope of practice at the beginning of the shift.
List 'unknowns' to be explored after your shift.	Alert the team leader if one of your patients has multiple care needs that are outside of your scope of practice.
Review lists regularly during your shift so that you are always aware of your responsibilities.	If you get behind in your care tasks, seek assistance as early as possible.

It is essential that you have reasonable and manageable workloads so that you can learn at your own pace. Make it clear to your team leader if your workload is too great or if a patient in your care has care requirements that are outside of your scope of practice. Explain that you will need support in many aspects of care and it would be more feasible to allocate you a patient where you need to seek support only once or twice during the shift rather than five or six times. Seeking support early rather than later is vital so that the team leader can reallocate workloads and put support mechanisms in place.

Learning through feedback

Seeking feedback from patients and their families and other health care professionals will help you to understand where your knowledge or care gaps may be. When seeking feedback, ask specific questions. Rather than ask, 'How did I go?', ask a specific question; for example, 'When I explained to you how the lock out system worked on the PCA (patient-controlled analgesia), was that clear or could I have done it a different way?' This approach should provide you with clear and constructive feedback to further your learning and allows you to pace and shape your learning as a GRN, as you can determine when you receive feedback and in what form.

Remember that all feedback is valuable, even if you don't agree with it. Reflect closely on the feedback and most times there will be something there that you can work with or from … even if it is to never provide that type of feedback when you are in a similar position. Think about why the person has provided the content of the feedback in the format that they did and how you will best respond to it professionally and objectively. Personal feedback that includes reference to things such as your personal lifestyle, culture and/or choice of friendship groups should not be provided and if negative feedback of this type is provided, it is a form of harassment. This should be addressed as being in breach of the NMBA's code of conduct.

REFLECTION: WORKING TO YOUR LEARNING CAPACITY

Individually, write a list under the headings 'Learning enablers' and 'Learning barriers'. Under the first heading, list what enables or makes learning easier for you. Under the other, list barriers that you are aware of that impact on your ability and capacity to learn. For example, when do you get distracted while learning? When do you feel bored with a subject area, or find it difficult to make sense of the material?

Learning enablers	Learning barriers

a   In your class group, and referring back to Table 8.2, discuss what strategies you could implement to ensure that you will learn effectively and efficiently as a GRN in the clinical area.

b   Role-play how you might communicate with your team leader that you need an adjustment in your workload to ensure a better capacity for learning.

HOW DID YOU GO?

Transition to practice as a GRN is learning focused. You therefore need to be very cognisant of how you learn best and under what circumstances. Use your shift planner and your self-advocacy skills to ensure that your learning is of a quality and quantity that best suits your needs.

8.5 Self-care and being a safe GRN

Sleep and **relaxation** are essential for you to become the expert nurse you wish to be. During sleep the information stored in your short-term memory is moved to your **long-term memory** so it is there ready to retrieve at your next shift. To be sure that you have stored information from your shift in your short-term memory, it is best to review your shift planner and any notes you made before leaving the clinical area. This process should only take one or two minutes but allows for reflection and reinforces the information in your short-term memory ready for long-term storage. Do not undervalue the need to sleep and **rest** in your early transition as a GRN. It is not just the physical demands of nursing that are tiring, the cognitive demands of the job will deplete your energy levels too (Donovan et al., 2021). Look ahead at your roster and plan how you will gain enough sleep and rest, as well as eat well and maintain regular exercise.

relaxation
Conscious periods of time where the mind can reset and rest.

long-term memory
Information that is stored and retrieved as needed over a long period of time.

rest
Sleep and quiet times to address and restrict fatigue.

When dealing with heightened work-related stress levels, avoid falling into the trap of short-term solutions, such as routinely eating non-nutritious foods, or regularly consuming alcohol, tobacco products or medications. Also, take on the mindset that 'work stays at work'. While you will want to reflect on a care situation or read about a medical condition to fully appraise yourself for the next shift, you should avoid worrying about something you did or said that you are concerned may have shown you in a 'poor light'. The aim is to provide the best care you can, hand over the person's care to the nurse on the next shift and leave it to them. The bottom line is to provide safe and effective care; you need to be well rested and cognitively and physically alert. If a patient knew that you were lying awake all night worried about them, they would not want you looking after them. A tired nurse who is questioning their abilities and ruminating about what happened yesterday or last week, is not in a strong position to provide quality care.

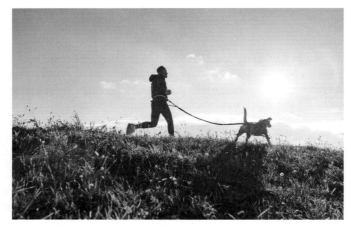

Source: iStock.com/Solovyova

Leave work in the workplace. Use your 'off-time' to reflect, recover and regenerate.

Gaining support beyond the health care team

It is a good idea to actively keep in close contact with family and friends. You may find it easier to bring your new family of health care professionals into your friendship network, which is very healthy and recommended. It is, however, important not to lose touch with those who knew you before you started working as an RN. They can tell you if they see changes due to a lack of self-care or see you becoming overly stressed or concerned. Seek professional advice (e.g. the clinical facility's counsellor, organisations such as Beyond Blue or mental health and wellbeing government websites) for any assistance you need to balance your work life with your personal life. Find exercise programs that fit around your schedules and plan out how you will meet your nutritional needs. There are countless opportunities for self-care (even for those who may live and work in regional or remote areas) and may be in the form of online apps, online support networks, 24-hour gyms, home delivery meals or planning out a weekly menu. Being fit and healthy is essential to be an effective and safe RN (see Figure 8.1).

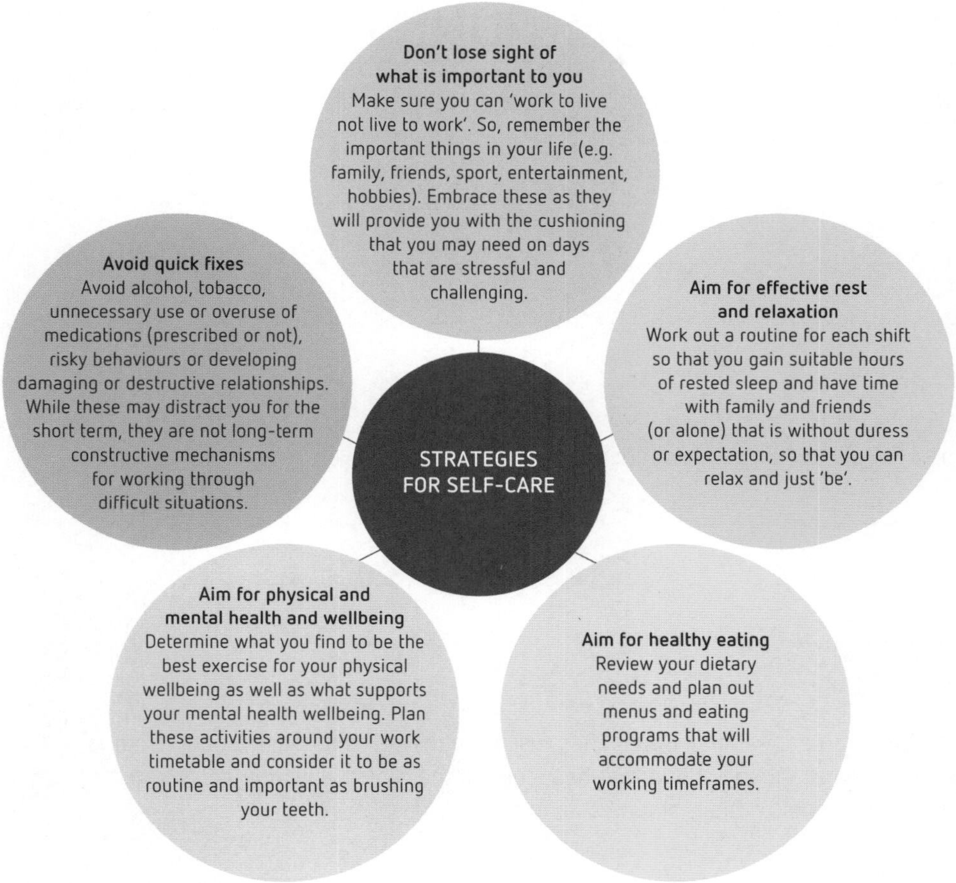

Don't lose sight of what is important to you
Make sure you can 'work to live not live to work'. So, remember the important things in your life (e.g. family, friends, sport, entertainment, hobbies). Embrace these as they will provide you with the cushioning that you may need on days that are stressful and challenging.

Avoid quick fixes
Avoid alcohol, tobacco, unnecessary use or overuse of medications (prescribed or not), risky behaviours or developing damaging or destructive relationships. While these may distract you for the short term, they are not long-term constructive mechanisms for working through difficult situations.

STRATEGIES FOR SELF-CARE

Aim for effective rest and relaxation
Work out a routine for each shift so that you gain suitable hours of rested sleep and have time with family and friends (or alone) that is without duress or expectation, so that you can relax and just 'be'.

Aim for physical and mental health and wellbeing
Determine what you find to be the best exercise for your physical wellbeing as well as what supports your mental health wellbeing. Plan these activities around your work timetable and consider it to be as routine and important as brushing your teeth.

Aim for healthy eating
Review your dietary needs and plan out menus and eating programs that will accommodate your working timeframes.

▶ **Figure 8.1** Strategies for self-care

FOCUS POINTS AND MOVING FORWARD

Think critically about where you see yourself as an RN because working towards those career goals is important to your professional development. Choosing positions that interest you and suit your lifestyle preferences will create job satisfaction; so too will ensuring that your workloads are achievable and that you can learn at your own pace and in your own way. Never underestimate the influence your general health has on your ability to learn and to work safely as a GRN. Make it a priority to have a flexible lifestyle that will accommodate your health and wellbeing needs and adapt to the requirements of your profession.

DISCUSSION QUESTIONS

1. Think about your scope of practice and the expectations of being a GRN. Discuss how you could determine a realistic starting point in your career progression.

_____

_____

_____

_____

2. Discuss the relationship between adapting your learning pace to ensure best practice for you as a GRN with being a lifelong learner.

_____

_____

_____

_____

3. In relation to professional boundaries, discuss how you could gain support from family and friends about something that happened in the clinical environment, without breaching privacy and confidentially standards and code of practice.

_____

_____

_____

_____

REFERENCES

Donovan, H., Welch, A., & Williamson, M. (2021). Reported levels of exhaustion by the graduate nurse midwife and their perceived potential for unsafe practice: A phenomenological study of Australian double degree nurse midwives. *Workplace Health and Safety, 69*(2), 73–80. https://doi. org/10.1177/2165079920938000

Fontaine, D., Cunningham, T., & May, N. (2021). *Self-care for new student nurses.* SIGMA.

Woolnough, H., & Fielden, S. (2017). *Mentoring in nursing and healthcare: Supporting career and personal development.* John Wiley and Sons Ltd.

USEFUL WEBSITES

Australian Institute of Health and Welfare (AIHW), Health workforce, www.aihw.gov.au / reports / workforce / health-workforce

Beyond Blue, https:// www.beyondblue.org.au

Australian College of Nursing, https:// www.acn.edu.au

Mental Health and Wellbeing, Queensland Government, https:// www.qld.gov.au / health / mental-health

Securing Australia's Nurse Workforce (2021), https:// www.acn.edu.au / wp-content / uploads / pre-budget-submission-2021.pdf

National Health Priority Areas, https:// www.health.gov.au / sites / default / files / australia-s-long-term-national-health-plan_0.pdf

National Women's Health Strategy, https:// www.health.gov.au / resources / publications / national-womens-health-strategy-2020-2030

National Men's Health Strategy, https:// www.health.gov.au / resources / publications / national-mens-health-strategy-2020-2030

SOCIALISATION AND PROFESSIONAL DEVELOPMENT

Learning objectives

Working through this chapter will enable you to:

1. argue that safe practice is not only that the patient is safe but that you are able to practice in a safe and supportive environment
2. examine the social dynamics of work environments
3. be actively aware of your health care environment so as to work effectively within cultural norms and professional expectations
4. cultivate professional networks by getting to know health care colleagues from a number of perspectives.

Introduction

socialisation
An opportunity to learn from colleagues how a clinical area functions.

The concept of **socialisation** has both positive and negative connotations. The negative suggests that you may be coerced or manipulated into conforming to the expectations of the clinical area you work in and becoming a clone of those around you. The positive connotation is that socialisation is the opportunity for you to gain an understanding of the culture of your clinical area and to grasp how the standards and codes of practice are applied in this clinical setting to facilitate safe person-centred care. In your graduate year your professional development is centred on what you learn and what you are exposed to in the clinical setting, so regardless of your perspective, socialisation opportunities will assist you in your professional development and your goal of becoming an expert nurse. It is how you respond to these opportunities and select what is best for your learning that is important for your practice.

9.1 Feeling safe and being safe in your practice

The need to provide safe person-centred care underpins all your practice as a registered nurse (RN) and you will be reminded of this constantly during your nursing career. It is equally as important, however, that you feel safe, both personally and professionally, while working to the Nursing and Midwifery Board's (NMBA's) registered nurse standards for practice. At no time should you feel unsafe and unable to practice safely. The context of **safe practice** covers many dimensions including working within your scope of practice to enable safe patient care, that the environment is safe and the equipment you are using will cause no harm to you or the patient. Organisational expectations should not place you in an unsafe situation due to unrealistic workloads or force you to work outside of the professional standards of practice.

safe practice
Working within expected standards of practice.

Socialisation and safe care

Support and guidance from the health care professionals around you are essential components to your successful and safe transition to practice as a graduate RN (GRN). This is often referred to as the socialisation process, where you are learning how to work within the routines and expectations based on the professional guidelines within the clinical context of care (Moradi et al., 2017). This guidance will be a great influence on the experiences you will encounter in your transition to practice.

You commence your nursing career with a fundamental knowledge base of the Australian health care system, an understanding of the common health priority needs of the people you care for and, in general, the expectations of the profession of nursing. Even though you are expected to practice independently, at many points in your first year of practice you will need to seek advice and support from those around you. Often graduates think that they will only need support when learning new skills and only from other nurses. But support will be needed at some point across all aspects of patient care, from clinical decision making, prioritising care, delegating care, managing the procedures of the clinical environment and working with patients and their families in demanding circumstances (see Figure 9.1).

Finding support within the interprofessional health care team

Do not think that the nurse team leader, your preceptor or the nurse educator are your only support personnel. Consider all the health care professionals in the team and other personnel in the health care area as primary support resources. Think critically and decide who could provide the most useful information to meet your needs at a given time. For example, dietary advice from the nutritionist, medication advice from the pharmacist or home care advice from the occupational therapist. Seeking the right advice at the right time will save you time and also give you the confidence that the information you have gained is accurate, safe and evidence-based. Having trust in the health care team is very important and will enable collaborative and safe practice. If you are in doubt of the advice you are given, however, seek another source (e.g. written, team leader, educator), as once you implement the action you are accountable for the outcome.

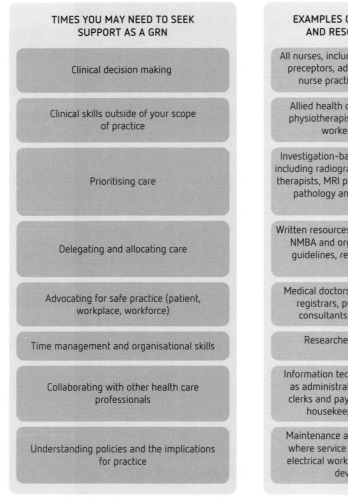

TIMES YOU MAY NEED TO SEEK SUPPORT AS A GRN	EXAMPLES OF SUPPORT PERSONNEL AND RESOURCES FOR THE GRN
Clinical decision making	All nurses, including clinical nurses, educators, preceptors, administrators, unit managers, nurse practitioners and nurse leaders
Clinical skills outside of your scope of practice	Allied health care professionals, including physiotherapists, speech therapists, social workers and psychologists
Prioritising care	Investigation-based health care professionals, including radiographers, sonographers, radiation therapists, MRI personnel and laboratory-based pathology and haematology health care professionals
Delegating and allocating care	Written resources in book form or intranet form. NMBA and organisational policies, clinical guidelines, research papers, government documents
Advocating for safe practice (patient, workplace, workforce)	Medical doctors, including interns, residents, registrars, public and private specialist consultants and general practitioners
Time management and organisational skills	Researchers / auditors who work in health care
Collaborating with other health care professionals	Information technology support staff as well as administrative personnel such as ward clerks and pay office, and services such as housekeeping and meal provision
Understanding policies and the implications for practice	Maintenance and engineering departments where service provision such as plumbing, electrical work and repairing of health care devices are required

▶ **Figure 9.1** Identifying and finding the support you need as a GRN

Knowledge of a comprehensive care plan

Having all the information you need to provide safe effective care is central to being an RN. The therapeutic relationship you develop with the patient and their family is based on empathy and will engender a domain of trust where they will feel safe to share information with you. The patient's medical history will provide you with details of investigations and other health care professionals' assessments, judgement and care management. If you feel, however, that you are being unintentionally or intentionally excluded from information and that you cannot provide safe care, you need to raise this concern. Be sure that the concern raised is always patient-centred, in that you cannot provide the patient with care if you do not have all the information.

Examples of reasoning could be that you cannot undertake a comprehensive assessment, your clinical decision making may be inaccurate, or your interventions may not meet the patient's priority needs. It is important to not address these situations from a position of personal limitation (e.g. I am just a graduate). If the behaviour is intentional, it then becomes a personal issue rather than a professional issue. Approaching these types of situations professionally ensures objectivity and provides you with a resilient approach.

REFLECTION: FEELING SAFE IN THE CLINICAL ENVIRONMENT

There are a number of factors that will add to your sense of safety in your practice. These include being supported and valued by a knowledgeable and professional team, being able to work within your scope of practice and having all of the patient's information available to you.

| Supportive team | Working within your scope of practice | Patient information |

Discuss these three points of safe practice in your group. Describe how these factors will enable you to feel safe when working in a clinical environment as an GRN.

HOW DID YOU GO?

You may think that providing safe care is a priority in your practice, but it is your safety that precedes all consideration of safe practice. If you are not safe when providing care, then it is highly probable that the people in your care will not be safe. Consider the support of the team and gain assistance if something is outside of your scope of practice. Make sure you are not being 'forced' to undertake skills and care that are outside of your scope, and be sure that you can undertake a comprehensive patient assessment so that decision making is accurate and valid. As a GRN these factors are fundamental to you being safe and being able to provide safe care.

9.2 Socialisation and your work environment

All work environments are different. This is due to the many professional, organisational and patient-care-based factors. It is also due to the people you work with, their values, priorities of care, experience and overall sense of purpose. You will see the different attitudes and behaviours of your colleagues and how this shapes the culture of the clinical area as well as your experiences as a GRN. As you work in your new clinical environment you will begin to accept the routines, behaviours and systems of the area as 'normal', and you may copy what you see around you.

belonging
A sense of connection and being accepted.

This perception of 'being on the same path' means you feel a sense of **belonging** and independence of practice. That is the central component of socialisation influencing the development of professional identity (Fitzgerald, 2020).

While this sense of belonging is important in your work environment, it is also important that you do not lose sight of yourself and your core values when providing nursing care. Being acutely aware of the workplace culture and the responses of your colleagues to the workplace will help you to understand the approaches in different

situational awareness
Awareness of the environment and the people who influence the environment.

situations. This **situational awareness** of how your colleagues relate to and influence the clinical environment is an important learning opportunity for you. Understanding the power of the nurse and how they can shape a situation with their behaviours and attitudes will inform your professional development and assist you in your

professional identity and perception of self.

The value of awareness in understanding socialisation experiences

The three levels of awareness that are commonly noted as important for nurses are self-awareness, **social awareness** and situational awareness

social awareness
Awareness of how you interact and influence others.

(see Figure 9.2). As a GRN, being self-aware will help you raise your awareness of your professional needs (Hodge & Varndell, 2020), your reactions and your ability to adjust your responses so that you can

ensure a professional approach to nursing practice. Social awareness provides an opportunity to think about how you interact with other people, and to understand the communication strategies you may be using and your ability to adapt those strategies to be a more effective communicator (Donovan & Forster, 2015).

SELF-AWARENESS
Awareness of your own needs, growth and ability to change.

SOCIAL AWARENESS
Awareness of how you interact and influence others.

SITUATIONAL AWARENESS
Wareness of the environment and the people who influence the environment.

▸ Figure 9.2 The value of awareness for the GRN

Both these levels of awareness are essential in how you respond and adapt to working in your clinical environment and the people around you. If you are unaware of your professional needs and responses, and you do not have the ability to adjust or manage your responses in the professional arena, you will not be in a position in which to seek out and develop your professional self.

Self- and social awareness are closely enmeshed with situational awareness, where the situation you may find yourself in will influence how you perceive yourself and those around you (Parse, 2018). Being acutely aware of the situation and how you and your team members fit within the health care environment enables you to take an objective view of unfolding events, the managed responses and your learning. This type of informed problem solving when working with a team of health care professionals facilitates a considered and focused approach. It will empower you to feel more in control and to understand the logical progression of care through a situation. Situational awareness takes practice and will improve as your experiences and understanding of the clinical environment and how those around you influence your practice become more familiar to you.

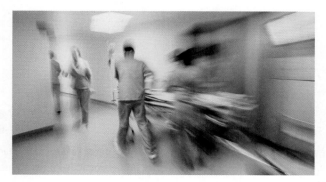

Source: iStock.com/vm

Situational awareness enables you to position yourself to ensure learning and best practice outcomes.

REFLECTION: UTILISING AWARENESS TO ENABLE SOCIALISATION SUPPORT AND PROFESSIONAL DEVELOPMENT

Select a clinical area of practice from your clinical placement experiences.

In your group, reflect on and discuss how using self-awareness, social awareness and situational awareness helped you gain an understanding of the people you worked with, and how this awareness assisted your professional development in the clinical area.

	Understanding your colleagues	Professional development
Self-awareness		
Social awareness		
Situational awareness		

HOW DID YOU GO?

Did you consider your colleagues from a number of different perspectives? It is important to not see health care as one-dimensional, as every health care professional has different perspectives from which you can learn.

9.3 Getting to know the health care team to enhance your professional development

In a busy ward your interactions with team members will be focused on the patient and their care needs, and as a beginner you will need to approach people you do not know for assistance on a regular basis. In general, the sooner you get to know the people you work with the sooner you will find who will be your best supporters, your 'go to' people and mentors. These people will be your earliest experience of socialisation and professional development.

The easiest way to expedite knowing who your 'go to' people are is to observe each staff member closely during handovers, their attitudes and behaviours in the general ward and how they engage in any case meetings, and also by attending any social activities that the clinical area may offer. Using these strategies to get to know your colleagues from a number of perspectives provides you with a valuable understanding of both their professional and personal selves. This allows you to be aware of what is important to your colleagues, their strengths and speciality areas of interest, how they like to be addressed and their preferences when being approached for support. Even knowing a person's sense of humour and their personality traits will provide you with more confidence as to when and how to approach them when seeking support.

Your ability to be socially and situationally aware is important as it enables you to observe and learn from the interactions and situations around you. Knowing which colleagues prefer to be socially active immediately gives you an indication of their preferred engagement style. Some staff, for example, are actively inclusive and will involve all disciplines of practice in the ward area by organising book clubs, walking groups, sporting teams or regular coffee mornings. Others may prefer to include only those of their own discipline in social events and yet others prefer to separate work from personal engagements completely. For example, consider the following case study.

CASE **STUDY**

GETTING TO KNOW YOUR COLLEAGUES – EXAMPLE

Jemma is a GRN who values friends and actively works to develop and maintain friendship groups. Jemma was pleased to learn that her clinical area holds a monthly social activity. She was even more pleased that each event was generally sports based, as she enjoyed sport and felt that it would give her something to speak to her colleagues about on the days after the event. The first social event was ten pin bowling and Jemma found that her team of four was supportive and outgoing. Jemma felt that the other teams were clearly made up of friendship groups who, while polite initially, were not overly friendly or encouraging. As the night progressed, however, she found that they did warm up to her and were complimentary when she bowled strikes or scored well.

At her next shift, Jemma worked with Ruby, an experienced RN who was at the bowling event and another RN, Sarah, who did not attend. Jemma easily fell into conversation about the evening and she and Ruby laughed about some of the more theatrical moments. Jemma felt that she had made a connection with Ruby, who told Jemma to 'call out' if she needed anything.

As Sarah was not at the event, Jemma felt awkward, but wanted to engage with her and commented that she missed a fun evening. Sarah responded with 'someone has to work' and that 'she's got enough to do without hanging out with work people'. Gemma felt put down and dismissed as not being serious about her job. She tried again and said that it was a really good opportunity for her to meet people from the ward. Sarah's response was that 'an eight-hour shift was long enough to spend time with the people in this ward' and walked away. Jemma was left standing alone and felt reprimanded for wasting time and went to care for her allocated patients. Throughout the shift she avoided Sarah wherever possible as she felt that Sarah did not think highly of her. Jemma knew, though, that she would receive positive responses from Ruby if she asked her for advice.

a   What are the disadvantages for Jemma if she only seeks support from Ruby?

b   How might Jemma adapt her communication to develop a professional relationship with Sarah?

HOW DID YOU GO?

Seeking support from only one colleague limits the advice and support that Jemma could gain. If she involved both Ruby and Sarah when asking for guidance, she would have greater opportunities to learn and to expand her scope of practice. It is worth persisting with developing professional relationships with all colleagues, as every member in the health care team will be able to provide support that will enhance the GRN's professional development.

While the case study is an extreme example, it is not unusual to work with very different personalities and people who have very different work ethics and social goals in your clinical area. Taking up any opportunity to engage with work colleagues is advantageous as a beginning RN, as not only will you begin to understand their perspectives on situations it will also help you to understand how they see themselves as a professionals. This does not mean that you should avoid or dismiss those who are not socially inclined, it means that you will need to approach them from a different perspective and be prepared to adapt your communication to be more aligned with their professional position (Donovan & Forster, 2015).

Creating your own social network

If you are in a clinical area where socialising is not regularly arranged or where there aren't a lot of opportunities to engage or even observe other staff members, start by meeting up with the other graduates in your clinical area. You can start by debriefing and sharing work experiences and expanding to other areas of interests and engagement. Work together on projects or learning activities that are expected of you so that you can share resources and ideas. This does not need to be formal and could be a 'walk and talk' opportunity or a relaxed coffee in the hospital cafe. Don't let the social engagements lapse as having this support structure becomes inherent in your networking and career planning. When you complete one gathering arrange the next one at that time. As you meet more staff on the ward, such as

social network
A group of likeminded people interacting on a personal basis.

second year graduates or as new GRNs join you, invite them along and expand the group. While not everyone will be involved, this is your opportunity to make lifelong friends and form your own professional and **social network**.

PRACTICAL APPLICATION: GETTING TO KNOW THE HEALTH CARE TEAM

In small groups, discuss ways of getting to know your professional colleagues from a number of perspectives. Using the figure below, note how you might get to know other members of the health care team. Consider this from a professional and social position.

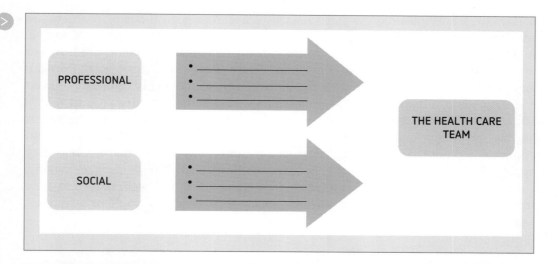

HOW DID YOU GO?

It may sound calculated to be focusing in on your colleagues, but understanding the people you work with is an important team building opportunity. Connecting with them on a professional level is a positive socialisation learning experience.

9.4 Professional development and your work environment

Understandably, your clinical expertise will develop and be influenced by your first RN role. Your expertise will increase with the differing patient care needs and the growing expectations of responsibility, which will propel you towards autonomous practice. While this may seem like a very ad hoc method of learning, determined only by what comes your way, if you have a definite plan or goal, you can make the most of these clinical experiences to grow your career towards your professional goals. For example, offer to care for patients with different conditions and health care needs so as to quickly expand your scope of practice and engage with specialised nurses and other members of the collaborative team in discussions about the people in your care to learn from their clinical experiences and expertise. Using every opportunity to expand your clinical experiences places you in control of how you are moving towards your career goal.

Learning by observing

It is of course important to remember that it is not only your clinical skills expertise but also your expanding theoretical knowledge and your professional attitudes and behaviours, that will progress you towards your career goal. Industry partners are consistently looking for graduates who have strong communication, critical thinking, mentoring and leadership skills. These are the skills that enable collaborative teams to work together and to ensure that conflict and issues of communication breakdown are explored and resolved. You can learn about these 'soft science skills' by observing your colleagues and other health care professionals' interaction practices (Court, 2020). Watch how the experienced staff communicate with people in different circumstances and assess patient needs quickly and accurately. Also observe how they select and employ equipment that ensures quality person-centred care is provided and how they apply their breadth of theoretical knowledge to inform their clinical decision making. Learning by observing not only provides you with a platform of best practice to draw from, it also enables you to role-play vicariously as to how you would or would not work with patients to achieve positive patient care outcomes.

FOCUS POINTS AND MOVING FORWARD

Socialisation opportunities allow you to observe the interactive and problem-solving prowess of your colleagues. It is also valuable to observe how these health care professionals practice self-care and advocate for their own professional development needs. Recognising these strategies gives you a solid foundation for how you too can work towards your career goals without losing sight of your values and what you wish to achieve as an RN. Being acutely aware of career options and opportunities is the first step to envisaging your professional self as an RN and also to futureproof your nursing career so you can experience consistent job satisfaction and ongoing professional development.

DISCUSSION QUESTIONS

1. A GRN reports 'they were so tired at work that they were falling asleep on their feet'. Discuss how this level of tiredness leads to unsafe practice where both the nurse and the patient are at risk.

_____

_____

_____

_____

2. Describe a time when you have felt a sense of belonging. Analyse and discuss the key components that facilitates a sense of belonging and how you would apply that to your clinical setting in your graduate year.

_____

_____

_____

_____

3. Describe a clinical placement experience when the environment was very busy. Discuss how 'learning by observing' is valuable for the GRN in such environments.

_____

_____

_____

_____

REFERENCES

Court, J. (2020). *Communication as a foundational technical skill for nurses*. Australian College of Nursing. https://www.acn.edu.au/nurseclick/communication-as-a-foundational-technical-skill-for-nurses

Donovan, H. & Forster, E. (2015). Communication adaption in challenging simulations for student nurse midwives. *Clinical Simulation in Nursing, 11*(10), 450–457. https://doi.org/10.1016/j.ecns.2015.08.004

Fitzgerald, A. (2020). Professional identity: A concept analysis. *Nursing Forum. An independent voice for Nursing, 55,* 447–472. https://doi.org/10.1111/nuf.12450

Hodge, A. & Varndell, W. (2020). *Professional transitions in nursing: A guide to practice in the Australian health care system*. Routledge, Taylor & Francis Group.

Moradi, Y., Mollazadeh, F., Jamshidi, H., Tayeheh, R., & Zaker, J. (2017). Outcomes of professional socialisation in nursing: A systematic review. *Journal of Pharmaceutical Sciences and Research, 9*(12), 2468–2472.

Parse, R. (2018). Situational awareness: A leadership phenomenon. *Nursing Science Quarterly, 31*(4), 317–318. https://doi.org/10.1177/0894318418792888

USEFUL WEBSITES

Australia's Health 2020: Safety and quality of health care snapshot, https://www.aihw.gov.au/reports/australias-health/safety-and-quality-of-health-care

Nursing and Midwifery Board of Australia, Registered nurse standards for practice, https://www.nursingmidwiferyboard.gov.au/Codes-Guidelines-Statements/Professional-standards/registered-nurse-standards-for-practice.aspx

PART 4

LEADERSHIP AS AN EARLY CAREER RN

Learning outcomes

1. Understand that all registered nurses, even beginners, are leaders in the health care system and know how to work within your beginning leadership role to achieve effective patient care.
2. Identify your leadership role and responsibilities within the collaborative interprofessional multidisciplinary team.
3. Apply a clinical decision-making framework to work within a chaotic health care environment.

Preamble

The Australian health care system is one of constant change where a persistent sense of urgency exists to meet the ever-changing health care needs of our society. Teams of clinicians and researchers are exploring medical problems around the globe, looking for answers to ensure a better quality of life for the people of Australia and beyond. As a nurse, you will be central to these changes with the expectation that you will keep up with new technologies and evidence-based practice, as well as being part of recognising the need for change while contributing to the research and education solution. Adapting to the changing needs of the people in your care and the changing health care environment will propel your ever-expanding scope of practice, and as a lifelong learner you will lead the changes through your knowledge, experience and discipline-specific application of nursing care.

In Part 4, you will learn about what it is to be a leader in a changing environment, how to fulfill the different leadership roles as a registered nurse (RN) and how being a lifelong learner will steer your scope of practice towards more complex knowledge and skills to that of an expert nurse.

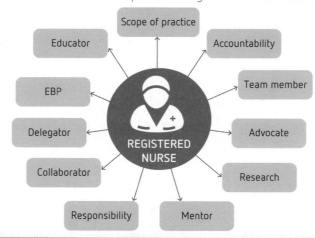

10 LEADERSHIP AND BEING A CHANGE AGENT

Learning objectives

Working through this chapter will enable you to:

1. explain the concept of leadership in nursing and how being a change agent is central to this role
2. use emotional intelligence to guide your leadership role
3. argue that all leadership roles must be actioned from within the registered nurse's scope of practice
4. recognise how delegation of care and advocacy are essential leadership roles for the graduate registered nurse to enable safe patient-centered care
5. implement evidence-based approaches to your role as nurse leader.

Introduction

Leadership in nursing has a long history. Most notable are Florence Nightingale, who led changes to practice to improve health care and reduce infection rates in injured soldiers of the Crimean war in the 1800s, and Lucy Osborne who brought nursing to Australia in colonial times. More recently, the importance of nurse leadership has been identified as an essential role of the registered nurse (RN), along with the obvious essential service role of the nurse, as highlighted, for example, during the COVID-19 pandemic. Nursing is a profession that recognises and drives the need for change. In this chapter, your role as leader will be clarified along with the expectations you will need to fulfill as a graduate registered nurse (GRN) in your first year of practice.

10.1 Leading as a newcomer in the health care environment

As a GRN, you may think that being a **nurse leader** is a role for senior nursing staff such as the team leader, nursing unit manager or the clinical educators. This is far from the truth as even though there are many different nursing roles and levels of responsibility

nurse leader
A registered nurse who provides a vision for change.

that an RN can hold, all RNs must be able to recognise the need for change and then lead to enable the change (Ferguson et al., 2020). And while often we think of leaders as those with booming voices, leadership does not need to be loud and coercive to be effective. For example, as GRNs you can very easily lead by role-modelling best practice attitudes and behaviours, such as effective hand washing, following medication check policies and working within professional boundaries. Also, leading by demonstrating a lifelong learning approach to practice that facilitates evidence-based critical reasoning and decision making, is another valuable strategy to demonstrate your leadership skills. An important quality in a leader is that they are committed to the leadership role and, as an RN, take **responsibility** for this role to ensure care is always current and evidence based.

responsibility
Adopting a duty to fulfill a role.

Roles and responsibilities of the GRN leader

What your leadership responsibilities are will depend very much on your RN role and the responsibilities that exist within that position. You therefore will have responsibilities related to duties and obligations of care and safety expectations that are specific to the role. You will be expected to fulfill your role and your responsibilities from a legal and ethical standpoint. For example, if your role is one of a clinician, then your responsibilities will align with direct patient care. If, however, your role is one of education, then your responsibilities will align with supporting knowledge and understanding. Both roles expect you to work within the Nursing and Midwifery Board of Australia's (NMBA's) standards for practice and codes of conduct, albeit from a different perspective. As a GRN you will most probably be working as a clinical nurse, so your leadership responsibilities are from that perspective. What is imperative is that your leadership responsibilities are always initiated from within your scope of practice.

Being accountable and responsible in your leadership role

Being responsible in your leadership role extends to bringing professional practice to your plan of care. As an RN you have a responsibility to provide safe person-centred care and to support your team members. Your input must be accurate and evidence-based, and you must be able to support your actions from your own learning experiences and evidence from the literature. Similarly, you must be accountable for the outcomes of the care provided and, as the leader overseeing and supervising the work, the consequences of the task. This is clearly seen in the leadership role of delegation where the **delegatee** takes responsibility for the care action, but the **delegator** retains **accountability**. This change in accountability is a primary transition expectation for the GRN, which needs to be understood in full and taken very seriously.

delegatee
A person who is delegated a task.

delegator
A person who assigns authority to another to undertake a task.

accountability
Being answerable for an outcome.

PRACTICAL APPLICATION: IDENTIFYING YOUR ROLES AND RESPONSIBILITIES AS A GRN

In a small group, and using the table as a guide, discuss the roles and responsibilities that are associated with a GRN when working in three different health care sectors.

Discuss the differences in the responsibilities and explain how these responsibilities shape leadership roles for the GRN.

Role as a GRN	Responsibilities as a GRN
Tertiary acute care respiratory ward	
Mental health community centre	
Rural hospital of 25-bed capacity	

HOW DID YOU GO?

During your discussions, you may have noted similarities in the care responsibilities. Responsibilities such as assessing the person's needs, listening openly and evaluating health care outcomes are all common for RNs. Could you dig deeper and identify how the responsibilities for RNs will differ in an acute respiratory ward to a mental health centre and to a small rural hospital? Recognising those differences will assist you in understanding your leadership roles in the different health care sectors.

10.2 Using emotional intelligence to guide your leadership role

As an RN you are automatically in a position of influence. Being very aware of how you may influence others with your interactions and being aware of each of the team members' preferences and needs is vital to being a strong and effective leader. Dismissing the needs and opinions of others leads to team members feeling undervalued and disrespected, which is a breach of the NMBA's Code of Ethics. An emotionally intelligent person is open minded and open to suggestions. They look for input from team members and take the input seriously. Decisions are not made without the needs of the team members taken into consideration, and the emotionally intelligent leader is trustworthy, honest and predictable. They are also decisive and prudent with information and consider all avenues before moving forward. As a graduate, you may find these expectations to be challenging; however, if you work within your scope of practice and within the professional guidelines set out in the NMBA's standards and policies, you will be in a safe space to begin your leadership role from an emotionally intelligent standpoint.

10.3 Leading within your scope of practice to achieve change outcomes

Your scope of practice is relative to your experience, knowledge and confidence. As a GRN you have had a minimum of 800 hours of clinical placement and have met the Bachelor of Nursing expectations of the Australian Nursing and Midwifery Accreditation Council to register as a nurse in Australia. This is no mean feat and with a significant amount of knowledge and experience under your belt you are entering the nursing practice as a beginning nurse leader. The narrowness of your scope of practice does not stop you from approaching your practice critically and ensuring that the people in your care receive evidence-based and safe care.

What is vital as a nurse leader is that you lead from a position of knowledge and understanding rather than from ignorance. As a leader you must ensure a comprehensive understanding of a situation by speaking to all persons and stakeholders involved and gaining information about previous experiences in the area. It is important as a leader to understand if your team members share your concerns or if there is ambivalence and acceptance of the status quo. Listening to the input of others means that you will learn from any barriers they may have met previously and ensures your team members feel valued and listened to. This new interest and vigour in the clinical area will encourage the team to come up with novel and creative ways to address an issue or to move towards a goal or vision (see Figure 10.1).

As a leader you must be committed to your role and any change that you may see as necessary. Your commitment must be shared with all members of the team, as you invite others to be part of your vision. Here your communication skills are essential in sharing your ideas and vision and encouraging members of the team to become part of the solution. Thinking about concerns and issues as problems to be solved removes the subjectivity and personal obstacles that you or others may have. Factors, such as feeling too inexperienced due to your **newcomer** status or being concerned that you may be part of or even the cause of the problem, hinder leadership. Addressing these barriers by seeking information, understanding what you need, looking objectively at the situation, and by gaining feedback from others so that your goals are based on knowledge and understanding, is the best place to start in your leadership role.

newcomer
A registered nurse who is new to the profession of nursing.

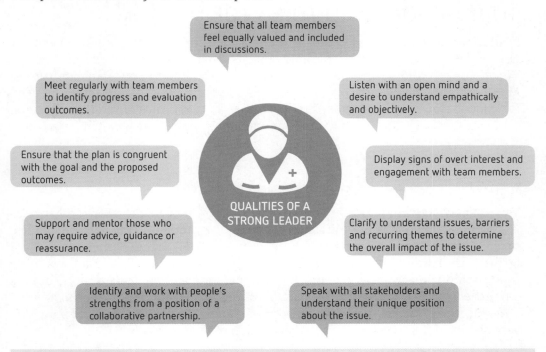

Ensure that all team members feel equally valued and included in discussions.

Meet regularly with team members to identify progress and evaluation outcomes.

Listen with an open mind and a desire to understand empathically and objectively.

Ensure that the plan is congruent with the goal and the proposed outcomes.

Display signs of overt interest and engagement with team members.

QUALITIES OF A STRONG LEADER

Support and mentor those who may require advice, guidance or reassurance.

Clarify to understand issues, barriers and recurring themes to determine the overall impact of the issue.

Identify and work with people's strengths from a position of a collaborative partnership.

Speak with all stakeholders and understand their unique position about the issue.

▸ Figure 10.1   Qualities of a strong leader

Gaining support from your mentor to develop leadership skills

As a GRN you will be looking for mentors who will guide and support you in your professional development as an RN. Your mentor will be invaluable in assisting you in your leadership role as a GRN. An effective mentor provides a professionally safe and inspirational environment where you will have opportunities for mindful reflection and expanded awareness of the clinical environment. It is this openness of thought and critical understanding that will help to unlock the leader in you. Seek a mentor who will not be afraid to challenge you to think beyond the obvious and assist you to find a space of professional growth. Also seek a mentor who will have the tenacity and the understanding of leadership to guide you from the beginnings of recognising the need for change through to where your colleagues and team members will also envisage and support the move forward.

10.4 Leadership roles for the GRN

Leadership responsibilities come in many forms for the RN, with the need for change driven by growing community needs, legal and ethical expectations of the profession and governmental positions. As a graduate your leadership roles are underpinned by your scope of practice and your ability to determine the need for change. You may be surprised to know that your RN roles of mentor, educator, advocate and delegator of care are four leadership roles that you will be working with as a GRN.

Mentoring as a leadership role

Very quickly you will find that you are in the position of mentor. Any person who is looking for guidance and direction may seek mentorship. This will include the people in your care and their family members as well as other members of the health care team. The important consideration is that you should always work from within your scope of practice and use communication skills that encourage a holistic approach to thinking and action. If you are asked for guidance in an area that you feel is outside of your knowledge or experience, then you should state this very clearly and not be drawn into a discussion of hypotheticals.

CASE **STUDY**

COMMUNICATING TO ACHIEVE AN EFFECTIVE MENTORING RELATIONSHIP

You are working as a GRN in a general practice (GP) super clinic. You were pleased that four new graduates were also employed and you formed a support group from day one. It is your fourth week in the clinic and one of the other graduates, Tracey, comes to you and appears to be very upset. She states that a patient had 'shouted in her face' insisting that Tracey had 'messed with her appointment'. Tracey says that she had no idea who the patient was but went with her to the receptionist to help sort out the problem. The receptionist pointed out to the patient that she had the wrong day and had now missed that appointment, and there were no more spaces until the end of the week. An appointment was made, but the patient was quite sure that Tracey was the problem and was making veiled threats to her of 'Just you wait until you're old', and 'You think you're so smart, but you're not!'

Tracey tells you that she feels she did not handle the situation well as she wasn't able to reassure the patient that she wasn't involved, and asks your advice. You recognise this as an ideal mentoring opportunity.

In your class group, determine the different types of language and communication strategies (verbal and non-verbal) that you would use to initiate an effective mentoring relationship between yourself and Tracey.

a   Discuss in small groups the value of mentoring as opposed to 'giving advice' in this situation.
b   What communication strategies (verbal and non-verbal) could be implemented to initiate an effective mentoring relationship between yourself and Tracey?

HOW DID YOU GO?

Mentoring opportunities arise many times and it is important that you are prepared to take on this leadership role when needed. Importantly, you should be confident that your role does not expand to being an expert and able to give advice. As a mentor you are enabling and guiding the other person to calmly review the situation from a number of perspectives so that they can learn from it and develop their own strategies. This approach is empowering and enables professional growth.

Patient educator as a leadership role

Many nurses will tell you that their greatest satisfaction is when they make a difference in someone's life. Being able to encourage, enable, support and empower a person to a level of wellness that they did not have before is central to patient-centred care. Knowledge is power, and when accurate assessments that identify a person's learning needs and knowledge deficits are used as a basis for change, then the nurse leader as an educator enhances the person's options and ability to make informed choices to move towards living a life of greater independence and enjoyment.

Advocacy as a leadership role

The 'call to arms' that the nurse must 'be the patient's voice' is fraught with complications for the GRN. Speaking out about something that is beyond your scope of practice or experience or outside of your professional role can be problematic. Speaking in error, without considering the situation as a whole, or understanding the roles and responsibilities of others, or the potential outcomes, can cause harm and breach the NMBA's code of conduct. Advocacy as a leadership role is one that demands complex thinking and holistic decision-making by the RN.

Before advocating for any person, policy or organisation, the RN should undertake a comprehensive assessment. All avenues should be explored by engaging with those directly involved, with others who may have had similar experiences, as well as reviewing relevant policy documents and literature that will accurately inform your decision. As a beginner, you may be surprised how much exploration is necessary to fully grasp a situation, but if you wish to promote and advocate for change, it must be undertaken from a position of full comprehension. If you are unsure of what your role of direct patient advocate may look like as a GRN, think about it from the perspective of ensuring that all patient rights, as outlined in the Australian Charter of Healthcare Rights, are achieved. The Charter's values concern all people in health care being listened to, being able to report concerns and feeling safe that their wishes are respected and valued.

Delegation of care as a leadership role

With the diversity of health care professionals and nursing personnel involved in health care, the need to delegate care has become essential to ensure timely and safe practice. The nurse leadership skills needed for the effective delegation of care are:

- accurate assessment
- effective communication
- open listening
- organisational skills
- persistence
- working within your scope of practice.

The GRN can struggle with the task of delegation. The reasons are broad but generally noted to be due to a lack of confidence in their ability to accurately assess patient health care needs and to delegate care to the most suitable person, being unsure as to the boundaries of their scope of practice and subsequent supervisory limitations, and a general belief that to learn they need to do everything (see Table 10.1).

For the GRN, the expectation is that as a nurse leader you will delegate care and supervise the delegatee safely and effectively from your first day of practice. Working with the NMBA's Decision-making framework and realising that while you delegate the responsibility of care you maintain accountability for the outcome can be daunting for the GRN. Being confident that your knowledge, competence and experience will

▸ **Table 10.1** Limitations GRNs have identified

Limitations GRNs have identified when thinking about delegating care
Knowledge deficit limiting their ability to undertake a comprehensive assessment of the patient's care needs.
Not knowing the delegatee's scope of practice or how to assess it.
Being unsure of their own scope of practice and are, therefore, hesitant to delegate as they are not confident that their supervision will be sufficient.
Lacking the communication skills to negotiate the task to be delegated with the delegatee.
Being unable to assess if the patient is stable or unstable and unsure if a person other than an RN can provide the care.
Feeling that they will appear 'lazy' for not providing direct patient care and meeting their allocated patient load.
Feeling worried that there will be unresolved conflict with the delegatee if the delegatee refuses.
Being concerned that harm will occur to the patient to which they will be held accountable.
Being unsure as to what, or how, to provide education to the delegatee.

enable accurate assessment of the patients' needs and the delegatee's capabilities, as well ensuring that your scope of practice extends to enable adequate supervision, education and ongoing support of the delegatee is paramount to meeting this complex leadership role.

PRACTICAL APPLICATION: WORKING WITH THE PHASES OF DELEGATION

Individually, go to the NMBA website and seek out the four phases of delegation in the Decision-making framework for nursing and midwifery. Read these carefully, making notes and being sure you understand exactly what will be expected of you as a GRN.

Identify the four phases of delegation. In your groups discuss how each of the phases will empower you as a GRN to effectively delegate care. Then discuss and describe what you will be accountable for as the GRN delegating the task.

Delegation phase	Effective delegation outcomes	GRN accountability

HOW DID YOU GO?

Systematic frameworks such as the Four Phases of Delegation are very valuable tools as they provide you with a step-by-step guide that ensures no practice care needs are missed or repeated. The complexity of delegation is supported by such a framework and facilitates an outcome where responses to questions about outcomes (accountability) can be logically and reasonably addressed.

10.5 Leadership through research and evidence-based practice

The move for nursing education from an industry-based training model to that of tertiary education was not just one of changing landscapes, the move was in recognition of the unique model of care that nursing offers and that nursing in itself is an independent and essential health care profession. As a professional RN, there is an expectation that you will work as a lifelong learner from an evidence-based approach to practice. Leading through quality and peer-reviewed evidence ensures that the nurse leader has the strength and authority to pursue health care goals.

The nurse also leads with the initiation of research by recognising professional issues or clinical dilemmas that need to be explored to attain quality patient care. As a GRN, you are in an excellent position to lead through knowledge and evidence-based practice and to recognise anomalies in practice. Your learning is recent and your ability to access up to date information and research outcomes and to critically review these from a position of applying theory to practice, places you foremost in the leadership seat.

FOCUS POINTS AND MOVING FORWARD

Leadership in health care is an expectation of all health care professionals, with the intention that all members of the health care team work together to bring about change that improves health care outcomes. As a nurse you will never stop learning and you will never work from a platform of yesteryear as it may no longer be relevant to your practice. To work effectively and in a team, everyone must be up to date with evidence-based practices to lead as a team into the future of health care and nursing practice. This approach to leadership through lifelong learning will enable collaborative respect between members and enable the highest quality of care and up-to-date practices to be achieved.

DISCUSSION POINTS

1. Discuss an incident where you noticed that an early career nurse brought about change during one of your clinical placement experiences. Describe the process that was adopted and how the outcome was measured.

_____

_____

_____

_____

2. Discuss how the role of mentor can lead to changes in practice in a health care environment.

_____

_____

_____

_____

3. Engaging in evidence-based practice is a leadership role that influences best patient care
    outcomes. Discuss this point.

_____

_____

_____

_____

REFERENCE

Ferguson, C., Newton, P., & Edwards, J. (2020). Clinical leadership. In E. Chang & J. Daly (Eds.), *Transitions in Nursing. Preparing for professional practice*. (5th ed., pp. 227–238). Elsevier.

USEFUL WEBSITES

Nursing and Midwifery Board of Australia, Code of conduct for nurses, https://www.nursingmidwiferyboard.gov.au/codes-guidelines-statements/professional-standards.aspx

Nursing and Midwifery Board of Australia, Decision-making framework – nursing and midwifery, https://www.nursingmidwiferyboard.gov.au/codes-guidelines-statements/frameworks.aspx

Nursing and Midwifery Board of Australia, Code of ethics, https://www.nursingmidwiferyboard.gov.au/codes-guidelines-statements/professional-standards.aspx

Nursing and Midwifery Board of Australia, Registered nurse standards for practice, https://www.nursingmidwiferyboard.gov.au/Codes-Guidelines-Statements/Professional-standards/registered-nurse-standards-for-practice.aspx

Australian Charter of Healthcare Rights, https://www.safetyandquality.gov.au/consumers/working-your-healthcare-provider/australian-charter-healthcare-rights

11 INTERPROFESSIONAL COLLABORATIVE LEADERSHIP

Learning objectives

Working through this chapter will enable you to:

1. value the collaborative environment as a facilitator of best practice
2. explain how support from the collaborative team assists the graduate registered nurse to develop a resilient approach to practice
3. identify nurses' roles and responsibilities within the collaborative health care team
4. advocate for the nurse as a collaborative leader
5. compare your responsibilities within intra- and interprofessional collaborative teams.

Introduction

The collaborative team is made up of a group of health professionals working together to support the people in their care. As a graduate registered nurse (GRN), you will find great benefit working in such teams, as the opportunities for learning and professional development are significant and only bound by your collaborative ability to engage with the team.

11.1 A collaborative approach to practice

Communication in a collaborative environment is respectful, demonstrates an appreciation for the other person's knowledge and experience, and is based on honesty and trust. To achieve this, team members must ensure that they clearly understand each other's position by using communication strategies such as active listening, clarification, and reflective paraphrasing and summarising. It is also important that each team member's non-verbal cues align with what they are saying, and that facial expressions and body language remains open and engaged. A **collaborative approach** to practice is not hierarchical, meaning that no-one is regarded as more important or more valuable than another. It is everyone's knowledge and experience that is imperative and all collaborative team members enter meetings with a commitment to seek out the evidence-based opinions and perspectives of all members, and to work with that knowledge as a team to establish a common goal and a holistic plan of care (Slusser et al., 2019).

collaborative approach
Professional practices and leadership within a team space where everyone shares knowledge to achieve common goals.

There are leadership roles, however, when working collaboratively. The leader in this context will generally be the health care professional who is the most involved in the person's care. This can often be the nurse (if, for example, nursing care is the primary care need, such as wound care or medication administration support), and while you will not be asked to take on this role in your early practice years, you should be prepared to do so by learning from and observing other health care professionals leading a collaborative team. All collaborative team leaders need to be able to put their own personal ambitions to the side and work towards a common patient-centred goal that is based on the recommendations of all collaborative team members (Hodge & Varndell, 2018). This attitude is fundamental to the collaborative team's success. All team members need to be accurate and precise about their professional role, and their professional knowledge and experience within their existing scope of practice, no matter how narrow. A collaborative team leader will encourage a collaborative approach to practice where shared decision making and professional deference is central to the interactions, regardless of who makes up the team.

PRACTICAL APPLICATION: WORKING COLLABORATIVELY

a   In small groups, describe your experience of a patient handover that you provided in your most recent clinical placement.
b   Individually, complete the table below to indicate if you felt you were 'collaboratively heard' by your group when you were describing your experience, then indicate if you demonstrated collaborative behaviours when others were describing their experience.
c   Then, in pairs, reflect on what was effective and what was not in the discussions and if changes could enable a more collaborative approach to teamwork.

Collaboration – perceptions and feedback	Y/N	Your input as a collaborative group member	Y/N
Did you feel heard by the group when you were speaking?		Did you listen carefully to all the group members when they spoke?	
Was there a sense of interest from all group members when you were speaking?		Did you take notes and display a sense of interest when listening?	
Were you asked to clarify key points?		Did you clarify points from the presenters?	
Were you invited to give your experience by group members?		Did you invite anyone to describe their experience?	
Were you interrupted by another group member?		Did you interrupt another group member while they were speaking?	
Was there a clear leader in the group who facilitated open discussion from everyone?		Were you the leader in the group?	
Were there one or two people who dominated the group descriptions?		Were you one of the people who dominated the discussion?	

11.2 The collaborative health care team

The membership of a collaborative health care team includes all health care professionals who are relevant to the person's health care needs. Importantly, it also includes the person in your care and their family and caregivers. Collaborative meetings may involve the whole team, part of the team or may be one on one. As an RN in a hospital environment, you will work collaboratively with the person (and family members) in your care throughout your whole shift. If you are working in a clinic, school or community environment, your

collaboration
Approach to teamwork where all members have equal input.

collaboration will most likely be during their appointments or visits, or any other contact you make with the person. The important point to remember is that working collaboratively is not just for when you are working with other health care professionals or other health care teams, it is an approach to care that must be employed at all times and in all situations.

Being a GRN in the collaborative team

As an RN you are immediately a member of a collaborative health care team. Even nurses working in the remotest areas of Australia work with a team of health care professionals ready to support patients and provide the best care possible. As a GRN, your first year of practice is a time of great change and provides endless opportunities for learning and career development, and regardless of your inexperience, you will be expected to contribute when different aspects of patient care needs are discussed. This is fundamental to your role within the health care team and as a health care professional. You will be engaging with patients and their families, initiating and contributing to one-on-one interactions with other health care professionals as well as specific nursing care discussions, and all demand a collaborative approach to practice. It is essential, therefore, that you learn the fundamental skills of being a collaborative team member and leader and develop these skills as part of your expanding scope of practice and responsibilities as a lifelong learner.

11.3 RN roles and responsibilities within the collaborative team

Working collaboratively is not a passive role and not for someone who is happy to sit back and let everyone else do the work. As an RN in the collaborative team, your role is to identify the priority nursing care needs of the person in your care and express those clearly and concisely, while also listening openly and respectfully to the other members of the health care team's discipline-specific recommendations for best practice (Queensland Health, 2019). It is with an attitude of overt acceptance and respect for the other team members' opinions and recommendations that the collaborative team can work towards a common goal that is transdisciplinary by nature and hence not bound by rigid professional rhetoric (Slusser et al., 2019).

PRACTICAL APPLICATION: UNDERSTANDING TERMS AND INTENTIONS

There are some terms that you may not be familiar with when reading nursing textbooks and journals. As a lifelong learner, you have a responsibility to seek the meaning and intention of all language relevant to your discipline. In the last paragraph, there were some terms that you may not be familiar with or may not be clear as to how these relate to collaborative practice.

Seek the definition of each of the terms listed in the table below, then in small groups discuss how these terms relate to the sentence in which it was written and how that relates to you working collaboratively as a GRN.

Term	Definition	GRN working collaboratively
Priority		
Passive		
Concise		
Overt		

Term	Definition	GRN working collaboratively
Transdisciplinary		
Rhetoric		

HOW DID YOU GO?

When you begin as an RN, you will find some terms, abbreviations and discipline-specific language is new to you and this may impede your ability to provide care to your patients. Be prepared to seek advice and do not think that you can check it later as understanding the term may be vital to meet the patient's needs. This activity gave you an opportunity to learn the definition of a key word and then apply it to a practice situation; that is, collaborative practice.

11.4 Being a collaborative team leader

All members of a collaborative health care team, including the GRN, have a responsibility to engage in a collaborative approach to practice. This includes working with the professionalism that equates to the role in which they are employed. An effective team leader will listen and work with each team member, seek to understand their strengths or areas where support may be needed and assist them to achieve their goal (Montano, 2021). An effective collaborative team leader will fulfill all these expectations, but also empower all members of the collaborative team to share their professional opinions and recommendations, while moving the team toward short- and long-term goals that align with the patient's preferences and priority needs.

Understanding the roles and responsibilities of each member of the collaborative team is essential so that reasonable expectations are placed on each member. This is particularly important for the collaborative team leader. As a GRN, you may find that you are unfamiliar with some of the health care professionals' exact roles and responsibilities in the clinical context where you work. It is important that you address this quickly so that when participating in a team meeting, you can demonstrate honest respect for the person's position in the team. It also provides you with the knowledge as to who would be the best resource if you needed advice or support in your clinical decision-making responsibilities.

PRACTICAL APPLICATION: HEALTH CARE PROFESSIONALS' ROLES AND RESPONSIBILITIES

In small groups, individually select one of the health care professionals listed in the below table. Using the internet, explore and identify their role from similar job descriptions and regulatory body expectations and align these with the contexts of care.

In your group, discuss the responsibilities of the health care professional based on the role and the context of care listed below.

Health care professional	Role	Responsibility
Speech pathologist working in a special care nursery		
Social worker working with people experiencing homelessness		
Psychologist working in a paediatric oncology ward		
Ophthalmologist specialising in cataract removal		
Nurse practitioner specialising in palliative care in aged care centres		

HOW DID YOU GO?

Having a very clear and concise understanding of the roles and responsibilities of each of the health care team members demonstrates your professional interest in them as health care professionals ready to achieve best patient care outcomes. Actively engage with each health care professional when the opportunity arrives. Ask informed questions and encourage all team members to be engaged to ensure that all aspects of the patient's needs are met.

11.5 Intra- and interprofessional collaborative teams

interprofessional
Across different disciplines of practice.

intra-professional
Within the same discipline of practice.

The terms intra- and **interprofessional** are associated with many aspects of the health care system, with teams needing to work collaboratively and cohesively to achieve best patient-centred care. From a general health team sense, **intra-professional** means within a discipline, whereas interprofessional is across disciplines. From a nursing perspective when considering intra-professional practice, the focus is on nurses working within the nursing discipline. Interprofessional practice considers all health care professionals working together from a transdisciplinary position (World Health Professions Alliance, 2019). This includes the discipline of nursing (see Table 11.1).

The breadth of health care professionals working in the health care sector is significant, and with roles that span clinical, management, investigative, research and educational areas, there is a lot of information for you to gain. How collaborative teams work together, regardless of being within or across disciplines, is fundamentally similar. Common behaviours include knowledge of each other's roles and responsibilities, adopting attitudes and behaviours of overt respect and value for the person as well as setting and working towards an agreed goal (Hodge & Varndell, 2018). Working collaboratively in teams that demonstrate these foundational principles is a valuable environment in which the GRN can learn and develop their nursing career.

▸ Table 11.1 Collaborative health care teams

Intra-professional team	Interprofessional team
A team that is bound by their discipline; e.g. nursing only	A team that consists of people from across different disciplines; e.g. nursing, medicine, physiotherapist, pharmacist, dental, psychologist

GRN support and the collaborative team

Being part of a supportive and highly functional collaborative team provides an invaluable learning opportunity for early career RNs. The constructs of support, respect and valuing each other's roles that is central to the collaborative team enables the GRN to grow their knowledge and understanding by listening and working with other members of the team.

One aspect of working collaboratively that you will value greatly is that of shared decision-making. As a GRN, you enter practice with a fundamental knowledge base, beginning levels of experience and early clinical decision-making skills. While you need to make clinical decisions independently, you are also expected to make them within your scope of practice, so if the knowledge and experience you need to make the decision is outside of your scope, you will need to include another health care professional to support you. You should also apply a collaborative approach to your clinical decision-making and include whoever is relevant to the decision and will be affected by the decision. This is always the person in your care and those health care professionals directly responsible for and involved in the person's care.

Another valuable aspect of collaborative practice for the GRN is that it facilitates and allows you to develop your communication skills as well as your ability to work collaboratively with others. You will feel empowered by those around you who clearly value your input and want to assist you in your professional development and career progression. It is with this level of support that the beginning RN feels safe to expand their scope of practice and develops a level of **resilience** that will advance their confidence and determination to ensure best person-centred practice is achieved.

> **resilience**
> The ability to take an experience and learn from it and use it to inform and grow your professional self.

Developing a resilient approach to practice and the collaborative team

Growing and developing resilience in a health care setting takes time and experience for the GRN. A collaborative team, however, will provide you with a safe environment in which to make mistakes and learn, to find your own rhythm and routine and to become the expert RN that you wish to be. Being resilient is having the ability to take an experience and learn from it and use it to inform and grow your professional self (Forman, Jones & Thistlethwaite, 2020). It is not about being able to absorb stress and distress and pretend it didn't happen. You are not meant to 'tough it out'.

For example, as a GRN your learning is significant and you will need to take a resilient approach when responding to the raised expectations, such as caring for a person whose medical condition you are not familiar with, or being asked to 'buddy' a student in your first six weeks of your graduate year. Ask yourself, are these expectations reasonable, is it achievable, am I gaining from these experiences or are they having a negative impact on my transition to practice?

Taking your concerns to a collaborative team member (usually the team leader), who will listen openly with an aim to understand your concern and how best to support you as a beginning RN, is a considerable step in developing your professional resilience. Approaching issues from a logical problem-solving position and using open and assertive language to describe and explain a situation, is an example as to how you, as a GRN, will be engaging in a resilient approach to practice.

FOCUS POINTS AND MOVING FORWARD

Collaborative practice is fundamental to health care and embraces key standards for practice such as the Australian Charter of Healthcare Rights and the Nursing and Midwifery Board's Code of Ethics. The centrality of respect and feeling valued propels the GRN into a professional realm of evidence-based practice and person-centred care. And it is with this level of support that you can transition into your clinical environment safely and confidently, while developing knowledge and skills that will enable you to work in the most chaotic of environments.

DISCUSSION POINTS

1. Health care professionals who work in a collaborative team environment feel respected and valued in their role in providing holistic person-centred care. Discuss this point.

_____

_____

_____

_____

2. Discuss why the collaborative leader could be any member of the health care team.

_____

_____

_____

_____

3. Discuss the relationship between a collaborative team and a resilient approach to practice for the GRN.

_____

_____

_____

_____

REFERENCES

Forman, D., Jones, M., & Thistlethwaite, J. (Eds.). (2020). _Sustainability and interprofessional collaboration: Ensuring leadership resilience in collaborative health care._ Palgrave Macmillan.

Hodge, A., & Varndell, W. (2018). _Professional transitions in Nursing. A guide to practice in the Australian health care system._ Allen & Unwin.

Montano, A. (2021). A concept analysis of interprofessional collaborative practice for community dwelling older adults. _Nursing Forum, 56,_ 413 – 420.

Queensland Health. (2019). _Interprofessional practice._ https://www.health.qld.gov.au/cunninghamcentre/activities/074

Slusser, M., Garcia, L., Reed C., & McGinnis, P. (2019). _Foundations of Interprofessional collaborative practice in health care._ Elsevier.

World Health Professions Alliance. (2019). Interprofessional collaborative practice. https://www.whpa.org/activities/interprofessional-collaborative-practice

USEFUL WEBSITES

Australian Charter of Healthcare Rights, https://www.safetyandquality.gov.au/consumers/working-your-healthcare-provider/australian-charter-healthcare-rights

Nursing and Midwifery Board of Australia, Code of conduct for nurses, https://www.nursingmidwiferyboard.gov.au/codes-guidelines-statements/professional-standards.aspx

Nursing and Midwifery Board of Australia, Decision-making framework – nursing and midwifery, https://www.nursingmidwiferyboard.gov.au/codes-guidelines-statements/frameworks.aspx

Nursing and Midwifery Board of Australia, Code of ethics, https://www.nursingmidwiferyboard.gov.au/codes-guidelines-statements/professional-standards.aspx

Nursing and Midwifery Board of Australia, Registered nurse standards for practice, https://www.nursingmidwiferyboard.gov.au/Codes-Guidelines-Statements/Professional-standards/registered-nurse-standards-for-practice.aspx

12 BEING A LEADER IN A CHAOTIC HEALTH CARE ENVIRONMENT

Learning objectives

Working through this chapter will enable you to:

1. navigate and prioritise nursing care in a busy and chaotic health care environment
2. apply the principles of advocacy to ensure a safe and care-focused workplace
3. employ a resilient approach to practice to enable learning and an autonomous approach to practice.

Introduction

The health care environment is pervasively and predictably changeable. Factors such as emerging technologies, changing patient care needs, workplace and workforce restructuring, and a raised expectation of time and attention from patients raises the health care environment to one of extreme busyness with at times chaotic consequences. As a graduate registered nurse (GRN), it is important to function effectively within your scope of practice in all types of health care environments. It is a valuable learning experience to prioritise the needs of the patients in your care and effectively advocate for them so that all their care needs are met.

12.1 Chaotic environments and the health care system

It is more common than uncommon to hear nurses describe their health care environments as busy, unpredictable and at times chaotic (Dahlkemper, 2013). And while this busyness and unpredictability reigns around the nurse, one constant remains, which is meeting evidence-based practice expectations and person-centred care that falls within the standards and policies as mandated by the Nursing and Midwifery Board of Australia (NMBA). As a graduate you might think that if you can master the clinical skills of nursing then your transition to practice will be easier. This is not always correct, and you will find that it is the soft skills to manage and work within demanding environments that industry partners are looking for in their graduates. The skills of being an effective communicator, thinking critically, being organised and working effectively as a beginning leader in a health care team are highly valued by health care recruiting teams. And while having the clinical skills are important to be an effective RN, it is those soft skills that are invaluable for you when working within a busy and chaotic health care environment and should be clearly recorded in your professional portfolio.

What does a chaotic environment look like?

All health care environments have the potential to be unpredictable and your clinical area can go from being an environment of overt calm to one of covert madness. All it takes is for a patient to deteriorate rapidly, one or two new admissions, one of the staff needing to take sick leave one hour into the shift, some faulty equipment or missing medication and suddenly the perfectly planned shift that you arrived to is but a memory. It is then that those soft skills come into play.

So, what makes for a **chaotic environment**? We know that it is unpredictable, so things happen that you didn't expect and didn't plan for. The chaotic environment becomes very fast paced as patients may need emergency care that is time sensitive, and with extra workloads, staff physically and mentally increase their pace of care to accommodate

> **chaotic environment**
> A health care environment experiencing unexpected and unpredicted change.

these. Typically, it will become noisy as there may be more staff needed to support, for example, a deteriorating patient where there are requests for investigations and other equipment. There may be discussions as to how best to solve the emergent problems and efforts to gather more people in the health care team who will need to be quickly oriented to the situation to ensure safe practice (Rucker et al., 2021).

Communication can become difficult when speaking becomes 'essential speech only', and often occurs when walking, writing and providing clinical care. Responses to questions are often brief and to the point and may be incomplete as the RN focuses on priority tasks. For the GRN, this environment may appear to be in conflict with what you have learnt as a student and impossible to comprehend. You may feel that your shift planner is a waste of paper and that the team has disintegrated into mayhem, and more importantly, that it is no place for a GRN.

REFLECTION: A CHAOTIC ENVIRONMENT

In small groups, discuss your experiences of a chaotic environment. Describe how you felt at the time, and how you found your space and could contribute to the changing landscape of the clinical ward area.

After these discussions, write a reflective paragraph about what you learned from listening to the members of the group as to how to work effectively in times of chaos.

HOW DID YOU GO?

Everyone's experiences are valuable, and discussing yours and listening to others enables you to vicariously learn from their experiences. You can then pursue and think about specific aspects of the experience so you can understand how it can inform and improve your own professional practice.

Being a GRN in a chaotic health care environment

First, never think that your presence in any clinical situation is not valuable. Just because your scope of practice is not that of an experienced RN, it does not mean that what you have to offer as a GRN is not essential. When faced with these situations, rather than stressing over what you can't do, think about what you can do. You can take vital signs and document, you can locate equipment, you can support family members and you can ensure that the environment is safe for everyone. That may include ensuring all rubbish is cleared away, a sharps container is easily accessible, any linen that falls on the floor is placed in the linen skip and clean linen is made available for when needed.

It is important that you continue to work with your clinical decision-making framework. This will enable you to assess the needs of the patients and health care professionals around you and give you a clear notion of what was achieved and what else needs to be achieved. Even though you have deviated from your initial shift plan, systematically and methodically you will emerge from the chaos having met the priority needs of the people in your care and supported those with emergency patient care issues.

Your initial development of your shift planner is very important when preparing for the unexpected. You must always allow yourself to have breathing space. This means that you should always allocate 'task free time' of about 10 minutes where possible between patient care needs (see Figure 12.1). As a GRN, these care intervals will provide you with a time window in which to reflect on care provided, prepare for your next clinical task where you may need to seek advice or support and, importantly when unpredictable change occurs, the flexibility to support those around you. Remember though that you cannot neglect the people in your care in an emergency situation. Assess and prioritise your own patients' needs, decide what must be attended to and what can be delayed a little, and become part of the solution rather than seeing yourself as inadequate or ineffectual.

Time	Patient 1	Patient 2	Patient 3	Patient 4
7 a.m.−7.20 a.m. Initial assessment, check documentation and prepare for breakfast.				
7.20 a.m.−7.30 a.m Space interval				
7.30 a.m.− 7.40 a.m. Prepare for 8 a.m. medications				
7.40 a.m.−7.50 a.m. Space interval				
7.50 a.m.−8.10 a.m. Give medications				

▶ **Figure 12.1** Shift planner example

12.2 Bringing about change as a beginning leader in a chaotic environment

It is when the health care environment becomes very busy and chaotic that the GRN really needs to draw from their leadership skills of patient advocacy and delegation of care. It is these two leadership qualities that will ensure that care is not omitted, and all staff can work in cohesion to achieve best practice outcomes, even in the busiest of times.

Advocating in a chaotic environment

Advocating for the patient in your care is central to your role as an RN and is clearly stated in the NMBA's standards for practice. Often patient advocacy is described as 'speaking for' the patient or being the 'patient's voice' (Zwilling, 2019). While this is noble it can disempower the patient by taking away their voice and replacing it with your own, which may or may not reflect the patient's wishes and be in breach of the Australian Charter of Healthcare Rights. A nurse misrepresenting the patient with incorrect requests and requirements can lead to inaccuracies in preferences and management, and ultimately patient frustration and more time and energy needed to rectify the situation in an already time-poor situation.

Advocating for patients in emergency situations, whose health may be deteriorating, demands nurses to be acutely accurate in their health assessment and seek support effectively and collaboratively. It is when the patient cannot speak for themselves, due to changes in consciousness or confusion, that the patient and the health care team rely on the nurse to explain what was observed and assessed prior to the deterioration. It is essential that you respond within your scope of practice and as a GRN that you seek advice early if you have concerns about your patient's health care changes (Mellor et al., 2017). This will enable both your input and that of a more experienced RN to give a comprehensive report to the team.

Advocating for a safe workplace

Advocating for a safe workplace is essential when working in a chaotic environment. It is imperative that all persons involved in the health care environment are safe, and in a fast-paced area this requires high levels of situational awareness where you are constantly looking for opportunities for unsafe practice and issues that could impact on the provision of safe patient care and a safe venue for staff.

SAFETY IN NURSING

WORKPLACE SAFETY ISSUES

Draw a floor plan of the layout of your last placement. Include all areas that you can recall. Identify where workplace safety issues were of concern/or had the potential for concern during your placement.

HOW DID YOU GO?

Being proactive is the best approach in health care. While most errors can be addressed with little or no negative outcomes, it is much better if errors are prevented from occurring in the first place. For example, supporting a person and their family members after a fall, or when incorrect medication is given or the wrong person is taken to X-ray, is not just inconvenient, it can be life threatening. Practicing situational awareness and remaining proactive is a good place to start.

Advocating for a safe workforce

A safe workforce is also imperative when working in a fast-paced and chaotic environment. To be effective, the nursing team needs a skill mix of staff who have the knowledge and skill to provide care for all patients even when an emergency situation occurs (Assi et al., 2019). As an RN, you and your health care team are lifelong learners and will be consistently ensuring that you are up to date in your knowledge and have the competencies in which to always provide safe, patient-centred care. As a GRN, your focus will be on expanding your own scope of practice by developing competencies and knowledge that move you towards being an expert and taking on a leadership role in times of chaos to ensure that all patients' needs are met.

12.3 Delegation and the GRN in a chaotic environment

Contemporary health care teams are made up of a diverse group of health care workers and professionals. The RN is central to and responsible for the delegation of care tasks to team members (Walker et al., 2021). One very clear stipulation made by the NMBA is that an RN cannot delegate care that is outside of their scope of practice. For the GRN this can become difficult if they are not sure of their scope of practice and can be more difficult in a chaotic and busy situation where they find it difficult to locate someone who can mentor and guide them in a pressured environment. In these situations, work to your scope of practice to ensure that the patient is safe and when assistance is available gain this as soon as possible to ensure that the care for the patient is completed.

The accuracy of your shift planner that targets from the beginning of the shift what care tasks can be delegated will assist you when you are feeling distracted by the noise and movement around you in a chaotic environment. Be sure to assess your patients at the beginning of your shift and from these, plan out the care that you will need to provide for your unstable patients, that which can be delegated and that where you will need some support. Set these plans in motion at the beginning of the shift by setting up the support timeframes and arranging delegation processes early. You can then focus on your patients' needs even when there are distractions from a busy environment.

Developing a resilient approach to practice in a chaotic environment

A resilient approach to practice is essential for the GRN when working in a busy and unpredictable health care environment. The resilient GRN will see a problem or an issue of practice and use this as an opportunity to develop skills and knowledge to overcome these issues (Irwin et al., 2021). To achieve this, you should draw from what you know and understand and move towards that which is unfamiliar. All clinical environments have a constant in relation to routines, standards and policies of practice and the roles, responsibilities and expectations of each health care professional's unique discipline. As a GRN, getting to know these factors of practice and those who you are working with will provide you with the foundations of your clinical area in which to draw from in times when the health care environment becomes erratic (see Figure 12.2). It will allow you the resources to work independently in practice while knowing who and where to gain support when needed, even in an environment of seeming chaos and disorder.

REFLECTION: A RESILIENT APPROACH TO PRACTICE IN A BUSY AND CHAOTIC ENVIRONMENT

Referring to Figure 12.2, list the key characteristics of resilience you were able to draw from when you worked in a busy health care environment during your clinical placement.

Which characteristics would you like to develop further?

Write a paragraph about how and why you think this development would assist you in your nursing practice when working in a busy and chaotic environment.

Discuss your reasoning with your classmates.

HOW DID YOU GO?

Were you able to pinpoint a characteristic of resilience that you wanted to develop to improve your practice when working in a busy and/or chaotic environment? Why did you choose that particular characteristic? If you understand why you chose it, you can more effectively evaluate your professional development in this area of health care.

Learning in a chaotic environment as a GRN

As a GRN, you will be given continuous opportunities in which to learn and gain experience and knowledge. Ideally the environment is one where, as the GRN, you can work to your own pace, have support staff who can guide and respond to your learning needs and access avenues to reflect and debrief on your experiences. If the environment does become chaotic and staff are needing to focus on emergency situations, there are still many ways in which you can learn.

Self-awareness and implementing a resilient approach of objective problem solving in these busy environments is very important. Focusing on where you are and where your role sits within the context provides you with a sense of stability. Also, being situationally aware and considering the environment as an opportunity to prioritise health care needs allows you to look for gaps and omissions of care, and

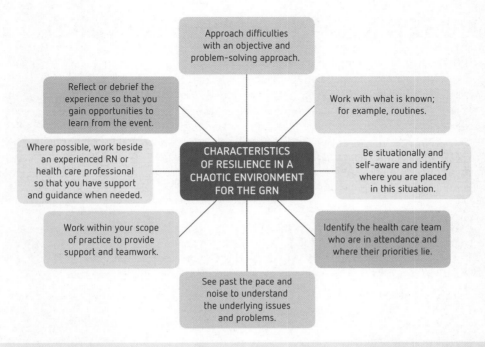

▶ **Figure 12.2** Characteristics of resilience in a chaotic environment for the GRN

places you in a position of learning from those around you. Be sure to utilise your clinical reasoning skills, by assessing patient needs and the environment carefully. Here you will be able to observe how the health care team's resilience in practice is working to meet the needs of the patients in their care.

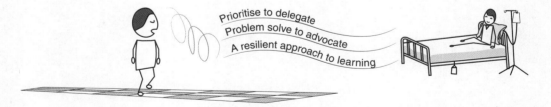

▶ **Figure 12.3** Moving forward in a chaotic environment with successful patient outcomes

FOCUS POINTS AND MOVING FORWARD

As a GRN in a clinical environment that may not be familiar to you, and with people you have not worked with before, you may find that knowing where to start when prioritising care in a busy work environment can be challenging. One thing that is predictable in health care are the common aspects of caring for a human being, while drawing from your professional knowledge and skills to support them. Being able to accurately and quickly assess and prioritise the health care needs of people in your care is central in your role as an RN. As you become more familiar with what is regarded as priority areas of care for your clinical area, the processes that must be completed for care to be provided, and the people who need to be involved in the care, you will manage times of rapid change more effectively.

DISCUSSION POINTS

1. Discuss how learning from experiences in all environments is important for the GRN's professional development.

2. Discuss the value of effective leadership within a chaotic or overtly busy environment.

3. Discuss how you, as a GRN, can advocate for a safe workplace at times of extreme busyness.

REFERENCES

Assi, M., Peterson, C., & Hatmaker, D. (2019). Workforce advocacy for a professional nursing practice environment. In B. Cherry & S. Jacob (Eds.). *Contemporary nursing. Issues, trends and management* (8th ed., pp. 232–250). Elsevier.

Dahlkemper, T. (2013). *Nursing leadership, management and professional practice for the LPN/LVN*. F.A. Davis Company.

Irwin, K., Saathoff, A., Janz, D., & Long, C. (2021). Resiliency program for new graduate nurses. *Journal for Nurses in Professional Development, 37*(1), 35–39. https://doi.org/10.1097/NND.0000000000000678

Mellor, P., Gregoric, C., & Gillham, D. (2017). Strategies new graduate registered nurses require to care and advocate for themselves: A literature review. *Contemporary Nurse: a Journal for the Australian Nursing Profession, 53*(3), 390–405.

Rucker, F., Hardstedt, M., Sekai, C., Mathabire, R., Aspelin, E., & Smirnoff, A. (2021). From chaos to control – experiences of health care workers during the early phase of the COVID-19 pandemic: A focus group study. *BMC Health Services Research, 21*, 1219. https://doi.org/10.1186/s12913-021-07248-9

Walker, F., Ball, M., Cleary, S., & Pisani, H. (2021). Transparent teamwork: The practice of supervision and delegation within the multi-tiered nursing team. *Nursing Inquiry, 28*(4), e12413. https://doi.org/10.1111/nin.12413

Zwilling, J. (2019). Multifaceted roles of the APRN. In K. Blair (ed.) *Advanced practice nursing roles: Core concepts for professional development* (6th ed., pp. 45–59). Springer Publishing Company.

USEFUL WEBSITES

Nursing and Midwifery Board of Australia, Registered nurse standards for practice, https://www.nursingmidwiferyboard.gov.au/Codes-Guidelines-Statements/Professional-standards/registered-nurse-standards-for-practice.aspx

Australian Charter of Healthcare Rights, https://www.safetyandquality.gov.au/consumers/working-your-healthcare-provider/australian-charter-healthcare-rights

GLOSSARY

accountability
Being answerable for an outcome. (Chapter 10)

acute care
Care of health problems that are short lived. (Chapter 4)

advocate
Someone who recognises and supports others. (Chapter 3)

belonging
A sense of connection and being accepted. (Chapter 9)

bullying
A situation where a person or group of people cause repeated and intentional harm to another. (Chapter 1)

change
A movement from one state to another. To transition into a different way of life. (Chapter 2)

chaotic environment
A health care environment experiencing unexpected and unpredicted change. (Chapter 12)

chronic care
Long-term care of health problems that are ongoing. (Chapter 4)

clinical guidelines
Guidelines that guide the nurse in the care of a patient. (Chapter 6)

collaboration
Approach to teamwork where all members have equal input. (Chapter 11)

collaborative approach
Professional practices and leadership within a team space where everyone shares knowledge to achieve common goals. (Chapter 11)

colleagues
Other health care professionals who nurses work with. (Chapter 6)

competency
Meeting expected benchmarks. (Chapter 1)

confidence
A sense of knowing that your judgement is correct and accurate. (Chapter 1)

conflict
A situation where there is a misunderstanding or misinterpretation of a message. (Chapter 1)

context of care
The place where care is provided. (Chapter 4)

cognitive saturation
A situation when the short-term memory is unable to store any more material. (Chapter 8)

continuing professional development
An expectation of learning (rated in points) that establishes the nurse's currency of practice. (Chapter 7)

cultural safety
Creating an environment where everyone feels safe, respected and valued. (Chapter 5)

data
Information in the form of facts. (Chapter 5)

delegatee
A person who is delegated a task. (Chapter 10)

delegator
A person who assigns authority to another to undertake a task. (Chapter 10)

diversity
The differences between people that make us unique individuals. (Chapter 5)

educator
A person who provides information and learning. (Chapter 1)

emotional intelligence
The overall ability to gain and apply knowledge and skills in relation to emotions. (Chapter 2)

emotional literacy
The skill to recognise, express and understand personal responses to situations and also recognising (reading) those of others. (Chapter 2)

empower
To encourage a person to feel more confident and able to achieve a desired outcome. (Chapter 3)

expert
A person who has high levels of knowledge and skills in a particular clinical area or discipline. (Chapter 7)

global health
An approach to health care that is worldwide. (Chapter 5)

health care team
All members of a team of health care professionals. (Chapter 1)

health promotion
Empowering people to take control of their health and wellbeing. (Chapter 5)

identity
How a person sees themselves. A person's identify gives purpose and meaning in their life. (Chapter 1)

imposter syndrome
A time where you doubt yourself and feel that you do not have the skills or abilities to deal with a situation. (Chapter 2)

interprofessional
Across different disciplines of practice. (Chapter 11)

intra-professional
Within the same discipline of practice. (Chapter 11)

ISBAR
A mnemonic tool that can be used in any form of clinical handover, which stands for introduction, situation, background, assessment, response/requirement. (Chapter 6)

leadership
An approach to nursing practice that influences others to bring about change. (Chapter 5)

learning
An event where information is applied to previous knowledge. (Chapter 8)

lifelong learner
A person who independently seeks knowledge and information. A perpetual learner. (Chapter 2)

lifelong learning
Learning that is motivated by an intrinsic desire to gain knowledge for both personal and professional reasons. (Chapter 2)

long-term memory
Information that is stored and retrieved as needed over a long period of time. (Chapter 8)

mentor
A person who guides or directs another. (Chapter 8)

National Health Priority Areas
Priority health care areas identified as significant for the Australian population. (Chapter 4)

networks
A grouping of like-minded people who support each other. (Chapter 6)

newcomer
A registered nurse who is new to the profession of nursing. (Chapter 10)

nurse leader
A registered nurse who provides a vision for change. (Chapter 10)

personal identity
How a person sees themselves in their everyday non-professional role. (Chapter 2)

portfolio
A file or compendium that stores experiences for the nurse in their growth and development as a professional. (Chapter 7)

practice readiness
Having the knowledge and skills to practice as a registered nurse. (Chapter 1)

primary level of care
The first point of contact with a health care professional. (Chapter 4)

tertiary level of care
Includes the highest-level medical, nursing and allied health specialist care and high-end investigative procedures and treatments. (Chapter 4)

primary prevention
Proactive interventions to prevent disease or illness. (Chapter 4)

proactive
Anticipating and acting on a need or situation before it occurs. (Chapter 7)

professional attitude
An attitude that exhibits the regulatory body's expectations when working as a professional registered nurse. (Chapter 1)

professional behaviour
Behaviours that exhibit the regulatory body's

expectations when working as a professional registered nurse. (Chapter 1)

professional boundaries
Invisible borders of practice aimed to protect both you and the person in your care. (Chapter 1)

professional identity
How a person sees themselves in their professional role. (Chapter 2)

professional nursing practice
Nursing practice that is within the regulatory body's expectations of practice. (Chapter 1)

promotion
Moving to a different level of expertise within a discipline of practice. (Chapter 7)

quandary level of care
Unique, highly specialised care facilities, such as transplant services. (Chapter 4)

rapport
A connection between people that is underpinned by empathy and understanding. (Chapter 6)

recency of practice
Nursing practice (rated in hours) that demonstrates that the nurse is up to date

in their clinical practice capabilities. (Chapter 4)

relaxation
Conscious periods of time where the mind can reset and rest. (Chapter 8)

rest
Sleep and quiet times to address and restrict fatigue. (Chapter 8)

remote
In this context, the measurement and extent of distance and space in Australia. (Chapter 4)

resilience
The ability to take an experience and learn from it and use it to inform and grow your professional self. (Chapter 11)

resilient approach to practice
Growing and developing from experiences, whether they are perceived as positive or negative. (Chapter 2)

responsibility
Adopting a duty to fulfill a role. (Chapter 10)

role stress
The level of stress that is experienced by a person in their professional role; often experienced by those who are new to a role. (Chapter 2)

routine
Behaviours and tasks that are so well practiced they become second nature. (Chapter 6)

safe practice
Working within expected standards of practice. (Chapter 9)

scope of practice
The extent of a nurse's ability to provide care based on their level of education and experience. (Chapter 1)

secondary level of care
Care that includes specialist medical doctors and more advanced medical imaging and pathology services in both a private and public hospital domain. (Chapter 4)

secondary prevention
Identifying a disease or condition in its early stages to prevent progression. (Chapter 4)

self-awareness
Awareness of your own needs, growth and ability to change. (Chapter 5)

self-care
A focus on your own needs to ensure best health outcomes. (Chapter 4)

self-manage
When a person can independently manage their ill health. (Chapter 4)

short-term memory
Information that has been recently stored for quick retrieval. (Chapter 8)

situational awareness
Awareness of the environment and the people who influence the environment. (Chapter 9)

social awareness
Awareness of how you interact and influence others. (Chapter 9)

socialisation
An opportunity to learn from colleagues how a clinical area functions. (Chapter 9)

social network
A group of likeminded people interacting on a personal basis. (Chapter 9)

support
Assistance that is provided to ensure that nurses can meet their responsibilities. (Chapter 1)

technology
Devices used to support health care practices. (Chapter 5)

telehealth
Health care provided using technological devices. (Chapter 5)

tertiary prevention
Preventing the escalation of an existing disease or condition. (Chapter 4)

transdisciplinary
A situation where different health disciplines' borders are blurred or crossed. (Chapter 2)

transferable
The ability to move skills and knowledge gained in one area to another clinical area or discipline. (Chapter 7)

vision
Imagining a concept or environment of change. (Chapter 7)

workforce issues
Situations that occur within the workforce; for example, communication breakdowns or staff shortages. (Chapter 1)

work–life balance
A situation where a person feels that their work life and personal life is at a point where one complements the other. (Chapter 2)

workplace issues
Situations in the work environment that impact on the ability of a nurse to practice professionally. (Chapter 1)

INDEX